Creating SOCIAL and EMOTIONAL LEARNING Environments

Amy Cranston, Ed.D.

Forewords by
Bryan Cranston and Michael Funk

Publishing Credits

Corinne Burton, M.A.Ed., *Publisher*
Conni Medina, M.A.Ed., *Editor in Chief*
Aubrie Nielsen, M.S.Ed., *Content Director*
Véronique Bos, *Creative Director*
Robin Erickson, *Art Director*
Seth Rogers, *Editor*
Tara Hurley, *Assistant Editor*
Lee Aucoin, *Senior Graphic Designer*

Contributors

Ernesto Durán, M.A.
Regional Lead, CDE Expanded Learning Division

Trisha DiFazio, M.Ed.
Adjunct Professor, University of Southern California

Kris Hinrichsen, M.A.T.
Teacher, Chinook Open Optional Program

Image Credits

Image credits: p.5, p.6 courtesy Amy Cranston; p.9 Lifetouch
Photography; p.11 Rick Smith Photography; p.32, p.70, p.93,
p.96, p.104, p.115 courtesy Ernesto Durán; p.34, p.55, p.78,
p.91, p.112 courtesy Kris Hinrichsen; p.85 courtesy Trisha
DiFazio; p.108 (top–both, bottom right) Scott Henderson
Photography; p.108 (bottom left) Annie O'Neill Photography;
p.122 TCM; p.136, p.137 courtesy Taylor Penny; p.138, p.139
courtesy Erica Fernandez; p.140, p.141 courtesy Jackie
Rotman; all other images from iStock and/or Shutterstock.

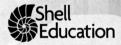

Shell Education

A division of Teacher Created Materials
5301 Oceanus Drive
Huntington Beach, CA 92649-1030
www.tcmpub.com/shell-education
ISBN 978-1-4938-8832-0
©2020 Shell Education Publishing, Inc.

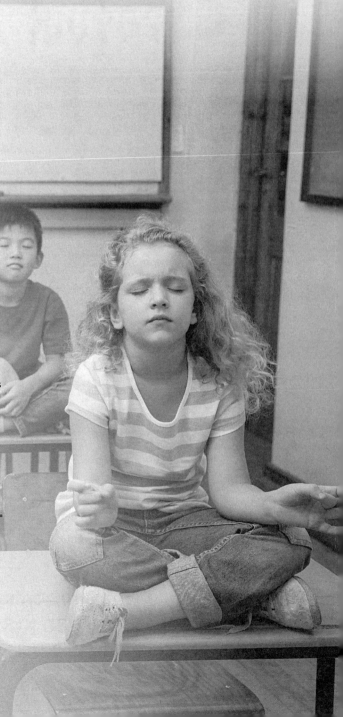

Table of Contents

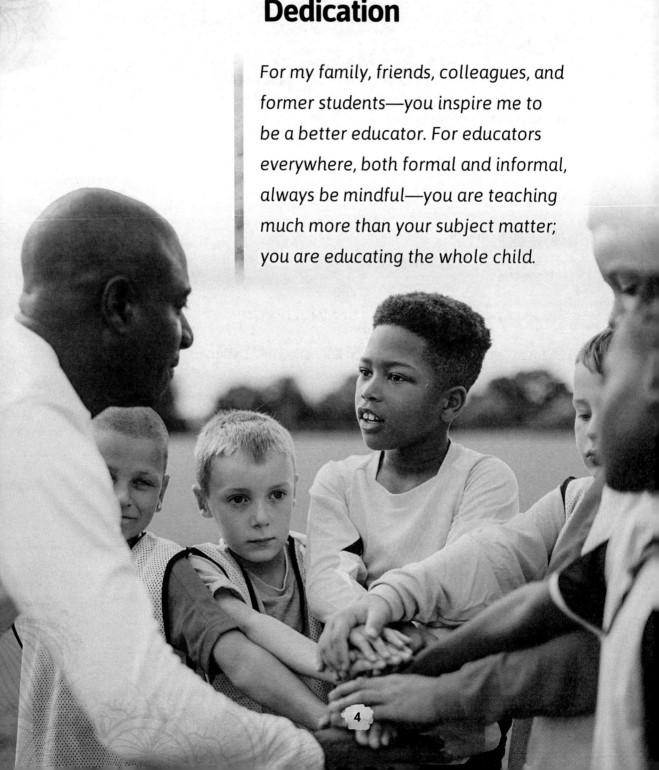

Dedication

For my family, friends, colleagues, and former students—you inspire me to be a better educator. For educators everywhere, both formal and informal, always be mindful—you are teaching much more than your subject matter; you are educating the whole child.

Foreword

As a young student, my grades were satisfactory, but my report cards often lamented such thoughts as *Bryan must start to focus more on his work*; *We need to see a more concentrated effort from him*; *Bryan just needs to try harder*; *Bryan needs to apply himself*; *Bryan is often goofing around and is disruptive*; *Bryan spends too much time daydreaming*. If I were a kid today, I'd probably be diagnosed with ADHD. But back then, the only diagnosis for my condition was that I wasn't doing a good enough job paying attention—as if I was purposefully disobeying my teachers. These comments, albeit coming from well-meaning teachers, tormented me like a bully, taking their toll on my social and emotional well-being, leaving me feeling inadequate as a student, and, to some extent, making me feel like I was stupid.

But then something changed and opened a whole new world for me. I've talked about this experience in my memoir, *A Life in Parts*.

> I was very fortunate to have two wonderful mentors in Mrs. Waldo and Mrs. Crawford, my fifth and sixth grade teachers at Sunny Brae Elementary. Neither of them was finger-wagging or textbook. They wanted their students to find their own ways to express themselves, and they encouraged me to explore performance. I learned that there were other ways to do a book report besides sitting down and writing the tired old "*Huck Finn*, Mark Twain's most acclaimed work, tells the story of the travails of a young man as he leaves his hometown seeking adventure...," blah, blah, blah. None of that. I could act it.

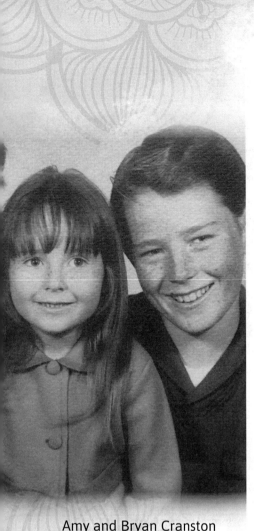

Amy and Bryan Cranston

My teacher-mentors didn't believe in the "one size fits all" mentality toward teaching, and I was the beneficiary of their philosophy—not just during those two short years in elementary school but for my lifetime. That realization made me see just how critical social and emotional learning really is for children. This aspect of education becomes the foundation for a happy and productive life. Without those teachers showing me a different way to learn, I don't think I would be where I am now. Their emotional support instilled a level of confidence in me that I hadn't felt before—that I never knew existed. Was it always there, lying dormant, just waiting for the right teacher or the right opportunity to express it? Regardless, that confidence grew. I suddenly felt empowered because I recognized that I was able to experiment in my learning and to value the lessons I learned from both my successes and my failures. I embraced trial-and-error and, in the process, developed a stronger work ethic. All of this, I believe, can be traced back to two caring teachers who saw a rambunctious kid and didn't disregard him or label him as a disrupter but kept turning him in a direction where he might eventually find himself. And he did. And I am eternally grateful to those two heroes in my life.

As an actor, it is imperative that I possess the skills necessary to tap into my emotions and to inhabit the emotions of the character I'm portraying. Paramount to this is the ability to put myself in another's shoes—to feel compassion, empathy, fear, regret, guilt, joy—the full spectrum of human emotions. For those who have experienced a challenging childhood, myself included, accessing your emotions can be a difficult and painful experience. The ability, or lack thereof, to access and manage your emotions can mean the difference between a successful adult life and a disastrous one.

It was important to me to write this foreword for my sister's book—to support her, of course, but also to support the hundreds of thousands of kids who I will never have the chance to meet. My siblings and I did not have an easy childhood. We found our way through our passions—mine for acting, my older brother Kyle's for social activism, and my younger sister Amy's for education. What I have learned from my little sister's book (I mean, *Dr. Cranston's* book) is that the whole-child approach to education is now embraced as a legitimate and effective method of teaching and learning. Teachers everywhere understand the power of helping students find and nurture their passions.

Bravo! Bravo, to all of you educators out there. You who have one of the hardest and most important jobs and who hold the well-being of future generations in your hands. I stand in awe of the work you do every day to provide all children with a well-rounded education and, like Mrs. Waldo and Mrs. Crawford did for me, give your students the opportunity to explore and *discover their passions.*

—Bryan Cranston
Father, Husband, Actor, Proud Older Brother

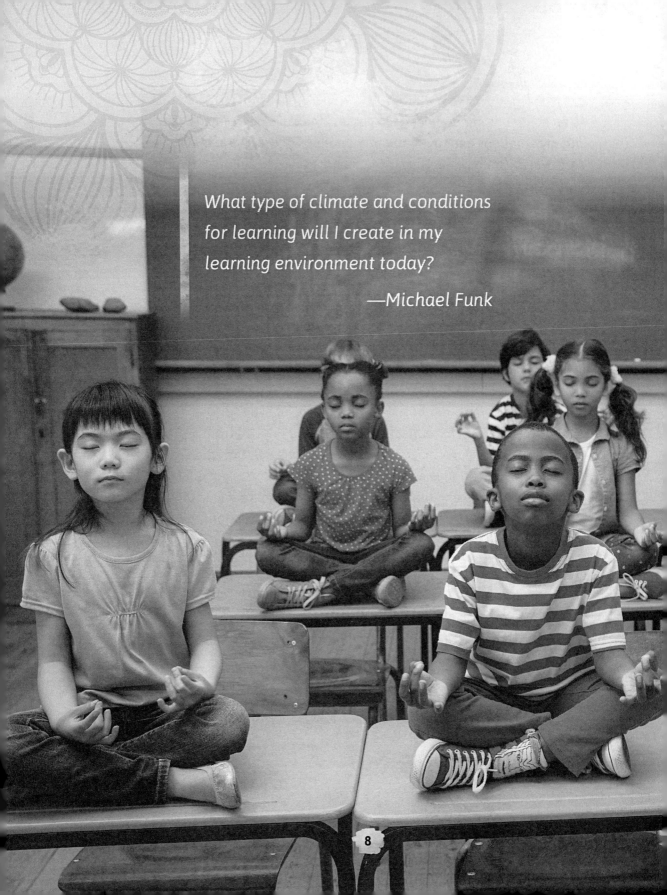

What type of climate and conditions for learning will I create in my learning environment today?

—Michael Funk

Foreword

When learning is referenced in a conversation about education, we are often referring to what a student is learning from the teacher, an expert in the subject. Not this time. **Learn**, the first *L* in the "3-L Challenge" of Social and Emotional Learning (SEL), represents the critical importance of an educator learning about themselves by asking, "How am I showing up in my classroom? How does my own awareness of how I am feeling on a given day influence how supported children feel when they are in my learning environment?" Social and Emotional Learning has to start with the adults. Too often I overhear educators ask: *What curriculum should I use to teach SEL on Tuesday at 2:00 p.m.?* Instead, that educator should be asking, *What type of climate and conditions for learning will I create in my learning environment today?* If we want children to develop self-awareness, resiliency, compassion, empathy, and many other SEL competencies, doesn't it make sense to start with the adults fostering those qualities and competencies in themselves?

For the past several years, I have referenced the contrast of transactional versus transformational leadership in California's expanded learning programs. I am not the first to use this framework. Many prophetic and provocative writers have described the transactional nature of our public education system and how this can be traced to the very design of the system in the beginning of the industrial age. We now understand that the presence of an authentic and caring relationship is the foundation for any system to move past transactions into transformations. In this context, I offer the second *L* in the challenge: **Lead**. At all levels of the education system, individuals need to ask themselves, *Am I willing to take the lead when others are waiting for someone to follow? Will I allow myself to become vulnerable and show up as my true self in order to grow trust in a fractured system? Am I willing to lead with compassion and empathy to foster a healthier climate and culture that will nurture the growth of social and emotional capacities in adults and students?*

In September 2016, I participated in a Systems Leadership Institute workshop led by Peter Senge, Robert Hanig, and Mette Böell. I was introduced to the "biology of empathy" and the "compassionate systems" framework coming out of the Massachusetts Institute of Technology. I must admit that some of the empathy exercises challenged my comfort zone, especially because I am a senior leader at the California Department of Education (CDE). It is not often you have the words *empathy* and *Department of Education* in the same sentence! I took a deep breath, understanding that this was all based in biological neuroscience. At least this gave me the footing to lean into the exercises. Fast-forward 36 hours—I had a profoundly spiritual experience that came out of the blue. This experience awakened me to the reality that, since coming to CDE, I had left a big part of who I am on the shelf. Somehow I assumed that the formal bureaucratic arena of education did not have the room or space for that part of me. So now to the third *L* in the challenge: **Love**. I left that conference knowing that I had to bring love to leadership and create the conditions for love to grow in our education systems for the adults who work in the systems and then, of course, for the children. A few months later, I was preparing for a plenary panel for a national conference. In that presentation, I acknowledged we were on the right path in addressing equity issues by recognizing that we are now moving the conversation from the *achievement gap* to the *opportunity* *gap*. What I then introduced was a more profound and deeper gap: the *love gap*. If our students don't understand and feel that they are loved and have the opportunity to love in response, then the expertise we offer will not close any gaps.

In short, what is social and emotional learning in its most distilled state? Love. This book is a wonderful resource to help us understand the context for this new emphasis and openness around social and emotional learning. It provides guidance for how each of us can impact another human for the better and find our own personal growth and transformation in the process.

—Michael Funk
Director, California Department of Education,
Expanded Learning Division

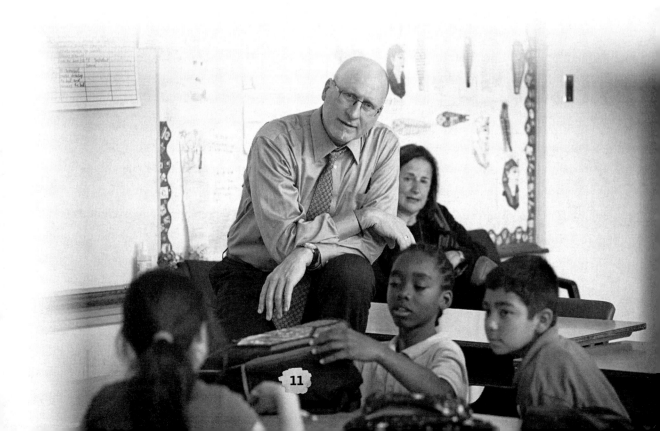

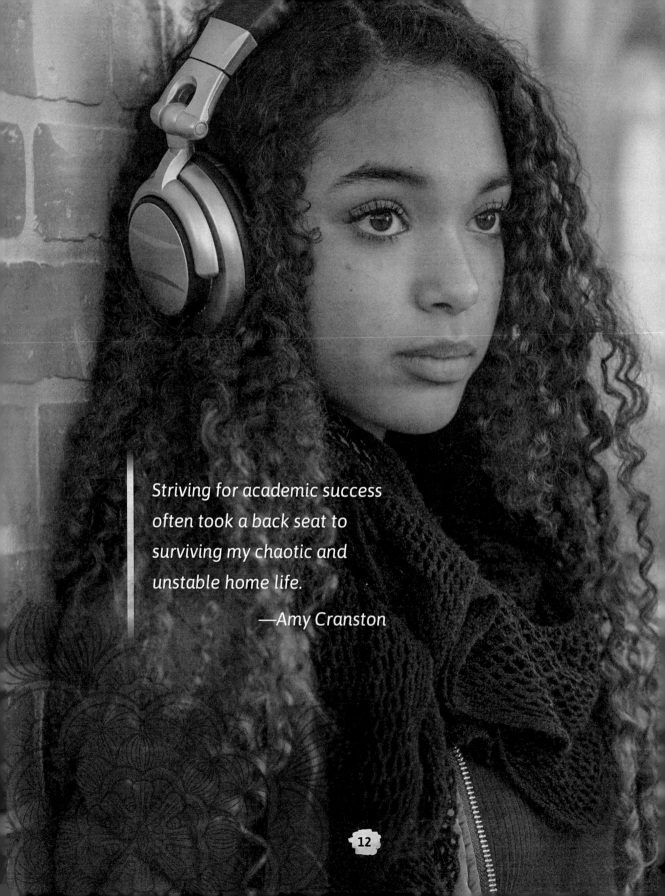

Striving for academic success often took a back seat to surviving my chaotic and unstable home life.

—Amy Cranston

Preface

Ever since conducting my doctoral research on social and emotional learning (SEL) six years ago, I have been fully immersed in the study of SEL. However, my interest in SEL dates back nearly 20 years to when I first began my career in education. I have always intuitively known this to be the most important part of teaching: being a caring adult in the teacher-student relationship, which was something I found to be missing when I was a student.

My initiation into the field of education was a nontraditional one. Teaching was a second career for me. After spending my first career in health care, I segued into teaching by sharing my professional expertise with high school students who were interested in pursuing a career in the medical field through a Career and Technical Education (CTE) program.

I was drawn to teaching at the high school level, perhaps because high school was the most difficult time for me when I was a student. I can recall a few fond memories of caring teachers in elementary school, but in high school—not so much. The emphasis was always on academic performance, and although I was a bright and capable student, I wasn't interested or engaged in school and did not see the relevance it had to my future. Striving for academic success often took a back seat to surviving my chaotic and unstable home life. As the daughter of a single mom struggling to put food on the table, college was not in the picture at that time.

As a high school sophomore, I started working at a restaurant after school. Although my academic studies may have suffered, I found the skills I developed through my work experience to be more valuable to my real-life education than school. For kids who have to work and become independent and self-reliant at an early age, school becomes less and less relevant to daily life. Sadly, I cannot recall a single teacher or administrator who took an interest in me as a whole person rather than just a seemingly unmotivated student. No one took the time to recognize or to inquire about the circumstances that propelled my disengagement from school.

Research tells us that dropping out of school is a process and not a singular act (Rumberger and Lim 2008). As I look back now, armed with the knowledge I did not possess as a teen, I was a textbook case of an at-risk kid destined to disengage and, ultimately, drop out of school. All the red flags were there, and yet they were not recognized by even one caring adult.

> So what does all this have to do with SEL? In a word— EVERYTHING!

What would have made the difference for a kid like me? Academic tutoring? Additional time allowed on tests? Disciplinary action for truancy? No, no, and no. The answer is support and nurturing of my social and emotional needs and development of social and emotional skills. Not the job of teachers and the school system, you say? Needs to happen at home with parents and family? Perhaps. But the reality is that educators are oftentimes better equipped to instill and cultivate SEL skills in students than are many families—if students are even fortunate enough to have an intact family and a highly functioning home life, which many are not. My message to educators is simple: Be the teacher *you* needed when you were young.

Think about the greatest character strengths you bring to your profession and to your personal life on a daily basis—these comprise your SEL skill set. How, when, and where did you acquire your SEL skill set? Did you learn these skills in school? Often, the answer is no. Most of us acquire skills such as teamwork, collaboration, and communication in the workplace. Commonly, these SEL skills are learned through life experience, trial and error, and learning from failure. Hence, a favorite anonymous quote: "Good decisions come from experience, and experience comes from bad decisions." Sometimes we learn from our successes, but more often than not, the greatest lessons are found in our failures. In his book, *How Children Succeed: Grit, Curiosity, and the Hidden Power of Character* (2012), Paul Tough praises the value of children learning from failure. Many educators struggle with this learning strategy as it appears to fly in the face of our desire to nurture and encourage success.

In speaking with successful adults, I have found that people cite myriad ways in which they obtained the essential life skills that they feel have contributed to their personal and professional victories. Often, they reflect on the SEL skills they obtained participating in sports, engaging in the arts, or through early work experiences, such as internships and community service. These experiences are how most of us learn SEL skills along the path to adulthood—often by accident.

But what if we could intentionally teach these skills to students as an integral part of their K–12 education? How much further along and better equipped would they be as they enter adulthood and embark on a career path? Can such skills be taught in school? And if so, how?

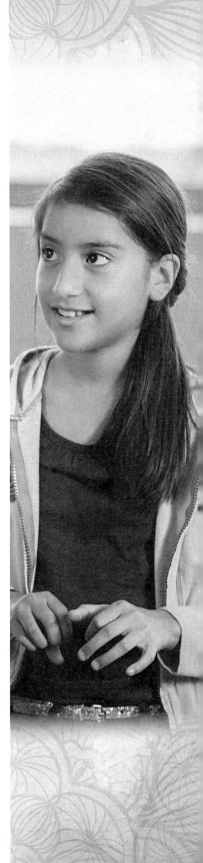

Acknowledgments

I would be remiss in my SEL skill set if I failed to acknowledge that I did not attain the experience needed to write this book all by myself. First and foremost, I want to acknowledge the vast contributions and inspiration for this project brought by my friend and colleague, Ernesto Durán. Together, we have jumped into the SEL waters with both feet, knowing that our younger selves would have benefitted immensely from a greater emphasis on SEL skill development both at school and at home. On the surface, it may appear that he and I come from very different backgrounds in terms of gender, ethnicity, culture, and age. However, our childhood experiences seem to mirror each other's in many ways. We also share a common bond in our desire to improve the life outcomes for all children, which is why we approach our daily work with students and staff from this standpoint:

> What do kids really need? What's missing? How can we fill that void?

This has become our passion and focus in the work we do together. Therefore, we always work as a team. In fact, *collaboration* is one of our greatest SEL strengths. Additionally, I'd like to acknowledge all the programs, staff, and organizations we have worked with over the years—thank you for your open minds, for your willingness to try new things, and for always having your students' best interests at heart.

A special thanks to Trisha DiFazio, who "discovered" me and encouraged me to take this journey along with the rest of the wonderful team at Shell Education. Thank you to Kris Hinrichsen, whose spotlights throughout the book show educators what SEL really looks like in the classroom.

Lastly, I want to wish a heartfelt thank you to all of the staff and students who participated in my research study, which served as the launch pad for this book. Individuals identified by first and last name are those I have a professional relationship with, and they are considered leaders in their fields. Therefore, unless a source is cited, their insights were the result of direct communications. To preserve the confidentiality of staff and students from specific school sites and programs, some remarks are attributed to pseudonyms.

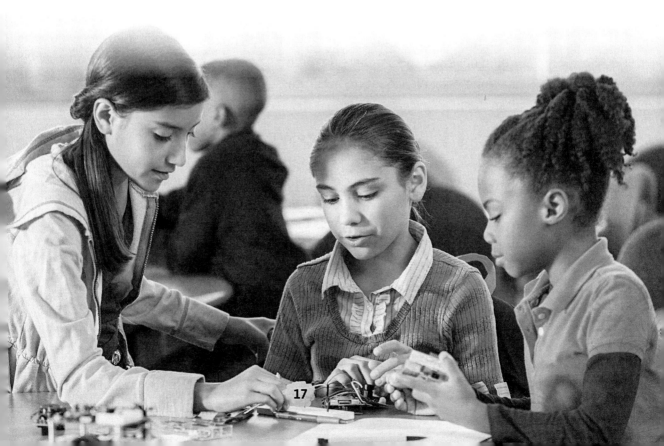

Is it really our job as educators to teach social and emotional learning?

Sadly, I write this book in the wake of yet two more tragic school shootings. Ten dead in Santa Fe, Texas. This on the heels of 17 dead in Parkland, Florida. When I attended high school, such a thing was unheard of. But that was a long time ago. Now, it seems we have become numb to such tragedies, and active shooter drills have become the norm. Improving school climate and safety is now a major focus in K–12 education. The Sandy Hook Advisory Commission, which includes parents who lost their children to that horrific event, expressed their support for teaching social and emotional learning skills in school, indicating their belief that implementing SEL programs would have positive impacts on creating safe and healthy school environments. We would be hard-pressed for a stronger endorsement than that.

According to the Sandy Hook Advisory Commission report (2015, 110–111), "Social-emotional learning must form an integral part of the curriculum from preschool through high school. Social-emotional learning can help children identify and name feelings such as the frustration, anger, and loneliness that potentially contribute to disruptive and self-destructive behavior. It can also teach children how to employ social problem-solving skills to manage difficult emotional and potentially conflictual situations."

By being able to identify and manage emotions and effectively resolve conflicts, we are more prepared to deal with life's challenges in school and beyond. And just as with academics, educators are often better equipped to prepare students with these essential life skills than are some families in our school communities. Yes, it is our job as educators to teach SEL skills to our students. I can think of no greater priority (Cranston 2017).

The 2015 replacement of No Child Left Behind (NCLB) with the Every Student Succeeds Act (ESSA) saw a shift in focus from standardized academic testing as the sole indicator of student success to a broader definition of what students need to be successful in school and beyond. With the implementation of nonacademic indicators of student success, as reflected in ESSA's verbiage, policy makers are acknowledging what most teachers have always known: kids need more than academics alone to become well-rounded, happy, and healthy (in every sense) students and adults.

This *whole child* approach to education is a welcome and long-overdue recognition of the value and impact of incorporating SEL as an integral component of K–12 education. However, educators now grapple with understanding exactly what SEL is and how it should be taught. What does it look like in the classroom? How can we leverage other educational environments in promoting SEL skills? How can SEL contribute to universally overarching goals, such as: addressing chronic absenteeism; improving school climate and family engagement; increasing student motivation and school connectedness; and strengthening college and career readiness?

The intent of this book is to remove some of the mystery around the elusive nature of SEL and share my firsthand experiences with implementing and cultivating SEL from a practical standpoint. The majority of my SEL experience takes place in the after-school setting, but you will find that many of these practices can be applied in other educational settings as well. Creating a healthy culture and climate for children that is conducive to fostering SEL is a goal we should all strive toward as educators.

As you delve further into your study of SEL, you will find plenty of research supporting evidence-based practices. My goal is to help you make the connection between research and practical application. Additionally, I hope to spark your thinking about how you look at SEL by broadening your understanding of where SEL lives and often hides, including in activities your students engage in every day.

It is my sincere belief (backed by abundant research) that SEL is a critical missing link in K–12 education. SEL is also a vital tool for enhancing equity and leveling the playing field for all students. ESSA brings a much needed opportunity and incentive to place SEL at the forefront of educational priorities for all K–12 students, particularly for underrepresented, at-risk students, such as those served in state- and federally-funded after-school programs and Expanded Learning Programs (ELPs). SEL is a cornerstone of high-quality ELPs, positioning ELPs to lead the way for implementing SEL practices in the K–12 instructional day.

Chapter One of this book provides an overview of SEL, including its historical roots and its contemporary iterations, supplying the background knowledge and context needed to establish a more concrete understanding of SEL. Chapter Two examines the role of SEL in addressing the current inequities and goals of K–12 education. Chapter Three paints a picture of what an effective SEL environment looks like. Chapter Four explores other avenues for leveraging SEL outside classroom walls. And lastly, Chapter Five examines the meaning of student success and the long-term impact of SEL on life outcomes.

My intention in writing this book is to help people who are new to SEL begin to grasp what SEL is, why it's important, and how to begin the implementation process in both your professional practice and in your educational environment. My concept of SEL takes the perspective that, just as with academics, all children have different interests and varied learning styles. This is not a one-size-fits-all approach to SEL programming.

Chapters begin with Mindful Moments to assess your existing knowledge and end with Points to Ponder to reflect on your evolving perceptions of SEL on the road to developing your professional practice. Included at the end of this book is a recommended reading list to further your research and a resource list to assist you in accessing implementation tools. This book is intended for all educators, both formal and informal and in a variety of settings, to help set the stage for effective SEL programming for student success!

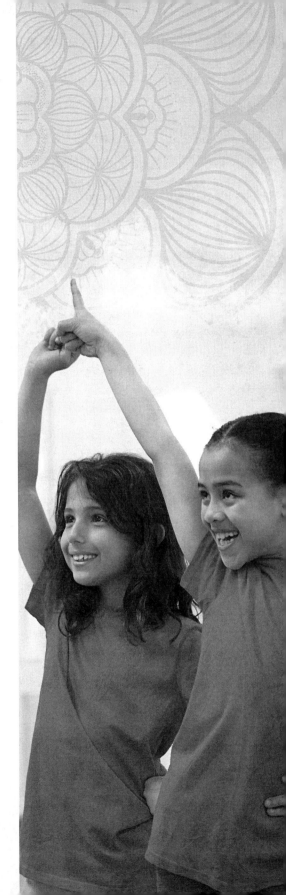

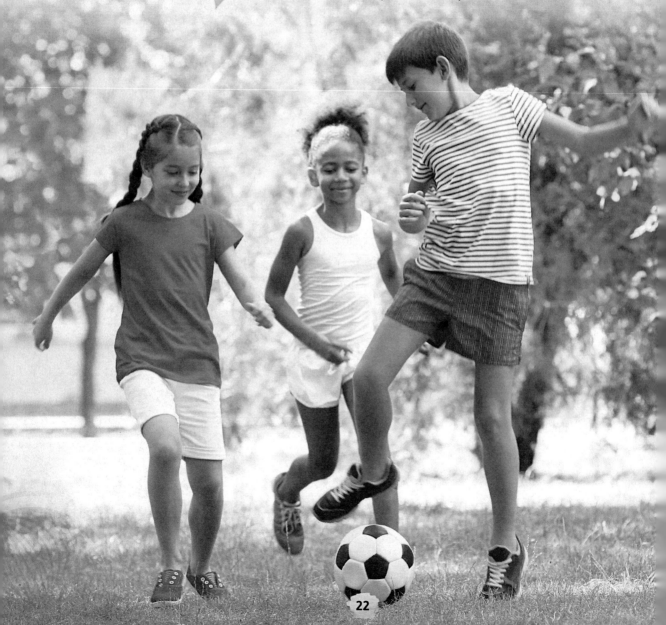

Social and emotional competencies aren't "soft skills." They are the foundation for all other skills. If we want a tolerant society . . . we need to teach the skills that create that society—the social and emotional [skills].

—Tim Ryan, U.S. Representative

Chapter One

What Is Social and Emotional Learning?

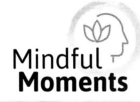

Mindful Moments

* What is your understanding of the term *Social and Emotional Learning (SEL)*?

* Do you agree or disagree with the following statements?

    » SEL is a fairly new concept in education.

    » SEL and academics are two unrelated skill sets.

    » SEL is meant only for very young children.

* How familiar are you with the following terms and concepts?

    » *EI/EQ*

    » *growth mindset*

    » *social agency/agility*

It seems the term SEL is everywhere these days. For many educators, this is met with a collective sigh of relief. At long last, we are talking about more than just academics and standardized testing when it comes to providing students with a quality education. To others, however, the buzz about SEL may be cause for concern. Is SEL merely a trend? Is it just the flavor of the month that will soon fade away only to be replaced by the next big idea in education? And then there are those who see SEL as nothing more than a shiny new name for an age-old concept. Indeed, an argument can be made to support any of these perceptions. Therefore, to provide some context and a deeper understanding, let's drill down into the historical roots of SEL, starting with the meaning of *intelligence.*

Measuring Intelligence

Early proponents of social and emotional learning include Howard Gardner and Daniel Goleman. Until Howard Gardner, a Harvard-educated developmental psychologist, published his theory of Multiple Intelligences (MI) in his 1983 book *Frames of Mind,* the field of education recognized only one form of human intelligence and only one method for measuring intelligence—the traditional IQ, or Intelligence Quotient. The IQ test sought to quantify the intellectual capacity of humans based on cognitive ability to solve a given set of problems. Gardner enlightened us with the concept that there is more than one type of intelligence. A decade later, Daniel Goleman (1995) expanded on Gardner's theory of multiple intelligences with his more specific theory of Emotional Intelligence (EI), later followed by his Social Intelligence theory (2006).

Gardner exposed how the concept of multiple intelligences impacts our entire education structure, which he refers to as the *uniform school.* The uniform school, Gardner explains, is one where all students are treated in the same manner, taught in the same way, and assessed or tested in a standardized format. While this seems on the surface to be a fair approach to education, Gardner argues that "this supposed rationale [is] completely unfair. The uniform school picks out and is addressed to a certain kind of mind . . . the IQ or SAT mind" (1983, 5). Gardner makes the case that, for those among us whose brains think and process information differently from the uniform school mind, "school is certainly not fair to you" (1983, 5). More recently, the uniform school mind has been referred to as students learning to "do school" as opposed to real-world learning, or what we often hear referred to now as twenty-first-century learning skills.

Gardner believed that "intelligences are not fixed from birth" and "how intelligence is defined, developed, and demonstrated will differ from culture to culture" (Elias and Arnold 2006, 37). If we fast-forward to 2006, we find this point echoed in Carol Dweck's theory of "a new psychology of success." Dweck introduced the concept of *growth mindset*, which is "the belief that your basic qualities are things you can cultivate through your efforts" (2006, 5). Conversely, a *fixed mindset* is the belief that one is limited to the intellectual

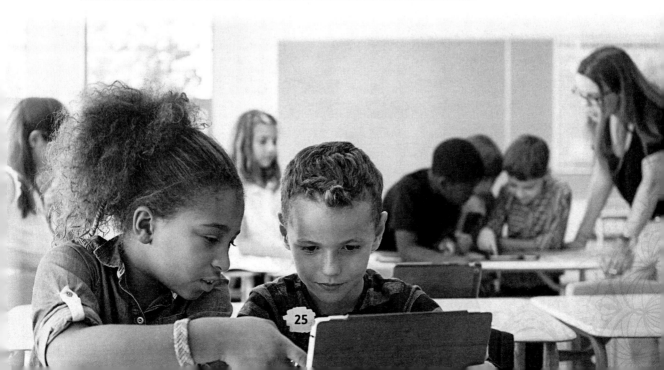

capacity with which one is born. Dweck believes that teachers with a growth mindset cultivate a growth mindset in their students. If the teacher believes in the student's ability to learn and grow through effort and practice—and instills that belief in the student—the student will indeed experience success.

Failing to adopt a growth mindset can have negative effects on students who struggle academically as well as those considered gifted. Dweck explains that students who are exceptionally talented academically are frequently praised and revered for their intellect. But such students can also be of a fixed mindset. These academically gifted students may be less likely to venture out of their educational comfort zones for fear of failure (Dweck 2006). Believing that only their intellectual capacity is of value can, in a sense, stunt their growth in other areas of development.

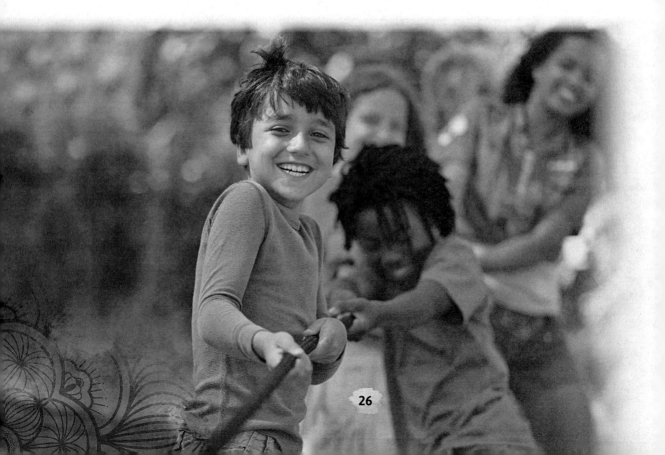

Emotional Intelligence and Social Intelligence

Goleman's theories of emotional intelligence and social intelligence gave rise to the term Emotional Quotient (EQ), a counterbalance to IQ. This "EQ" is another term heard bandied about as of late, not only in education but in the business world as well. Corporate leaders are on the lookout for employees who not only possess the technical skills needed to do the job but who also have developed the emotional intelligence required to work collaboratively and communicate effectively. Goleman, along with other scholars, views emotional intelligence as "the ability to perceive emotions, to access and generate emotions . . . to understand emotions . . . and to reflectively regulate emotions" (Mayer and Salovey, as cited in Elias and Arnold 2006, 36). Goleman contends:

"The emotional lessons we learn as children at home and at school shape the emotional circuits, making us more adept—or inept—at the basics of emotional intelligence. This means that childhood and adolescence are critical windows of opportunity for setting down the essential emotional habits that will govern our lives" (Goleman 1995, xiii).

This implies that if one fails to develop emotional intelligence during youth, it is unlikely they will learn to master these skills in adulthood. This in turn supports the reasoning of many employers that, while technical skills can be taught, continually developed, and improved over time and with experience, the same cannot be said for the ability to develop emotional intelligence through on-the-job training. Therefore, students with a solid foundation of emotional intelligence are positioned well to learn and grow, both in school and in the workplace, whereas students who excel academically but lack emotional intelligence are often ill-prepared for higher education and a successful transition into adulthood. A startling example of this is seen in a study of the KIPP (Knowledge Is Power Program) Academy.

Paul Tough analyzed the KIPP Academy in the South Bronx to evaluate what works and what is missing when it comes to supporting student success, particularly in older youths from underserved populations. In 1999, a group of 38 students of color (African American and Hispanic) from low socioeconomic backgrounds became arguably "the most famous eighth-grade class in the history of American public education" (Tough 2012, 49). This group of students had been recruited years earlier as fourth-graders by KIPP co-founder David Levin to attend his newly formed model middle school.

Levin's promise to the students and their parents was this: within the four years they attended KIPP academy, "he would transform them from typical underperforming Bronx-public-school students into college-bound scholars." Levin's model of an "immersive style of schooling . . . combining long days of high-energy, high-intensity classroom instruction with an elaborate program of attitude adjustment and behavior modification" appeared to pay off (Tough 2012, 49).

The students' academic achievement scores not only exceeded expectations but made history, garnering media attention as well as financial support for the KIPP model. However, these history-making students, the majority of whom made it through high school and into college, faced challenges that proved too much for most. "Six years after their high school graduation, just 21 percent of the cohort—eight students [of the 38]—had completed a four-year college degree" (Tough 2012, 50).

Tough describes Levin's devastation over the disappointing long-term outcomes, which manifested in not only the original group of KIPP students but continued in subsequent classes. "The whole point of KIPP was to give his students everything they needed to succeed in college. What had he failed to include?" (Tough 2012, 52). Levin's follow-up study on these students revealed something surprising—the students who completed college were not necessarily KIPP's top students academically. Rather, they were those who excelled in SEL skills, such as resiliency and social agency. These hidden traits appeared to be the secret sauce of student success. We may be familiar with the role resiliency plays in student success, but what is meant by *social agency*?

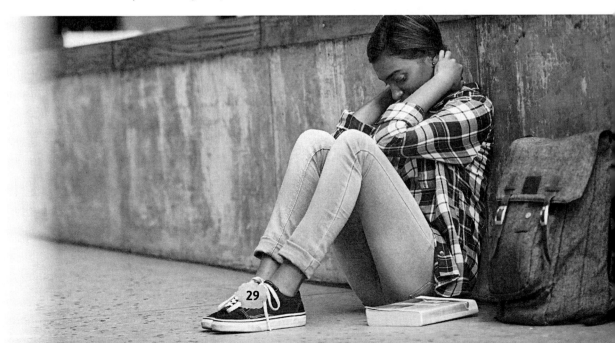

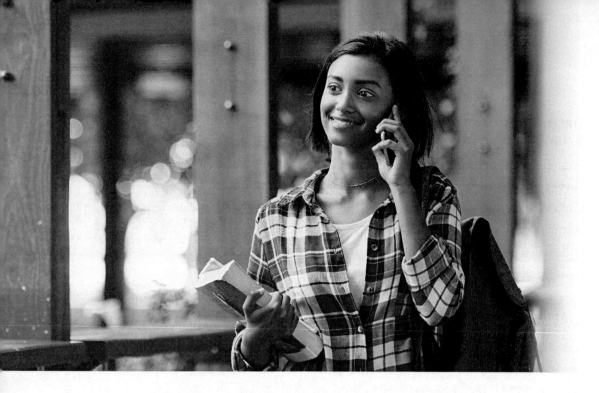

The terms *social agency* and *social agility* describe the ability to advocate for oneself and to successfully navigate through new experiences and unfamiliar environments. For example, the more socially adept KIPP students were those who possessed the ability to seek out professors and ask for help. Simply possessing the social awareness and confidence to reach out for additional guidance and support made the difference between persisting in college and dropping out.

What Levin recognized in these findings was that neither intense academic rigor nor adherence to strict rules and a highly structured learning environment were on their own enough to sustain long-term success. "For young people without the benefit of a lot of family resources, without the kind of safety net that their wealthier peers enjoyed, these characteristics proved to be an indispensable part of making it to college graduation day" (Levin, as cited by Tough 2012, 52). Successful students, despite adversity, displayed the ability to overcome failure and forge on with a positive attitude. They exhibited *resiliency,* or what Angela Duckworth (2016) refers to as *grit.*

Start from the Inside Out:
The Brain Science Behind Emotions

According to Eric Jensen (2009), humans are only "hard-wired" for six basic emotions: sadness, joy, disgust, anger, surprise, and fear. This concept was brilliantly illustrated in the well-researched Disney-Pixar film, *Inside Out*. Aside from these six hard-wired emotions, all others—humility, empathy, compassion, and gratitude, to name a few—must be learned. Jensen explains that for children living in poverty, accessing and managing these emotions is even more challenging than it is for their wealthier counterparts. For all people, but in particular those who have experienced Adverse Childhood Experiences (ACEs), such as the trauma and stress brought on by poverty, a condition called *emotional flooding* can frequently occur. Emotional flooding is essentially an emotion overload that overwhelms your psyche and affects your ability to process information and self-regulate, often resulting in the "fight, flight, or freeze" response.

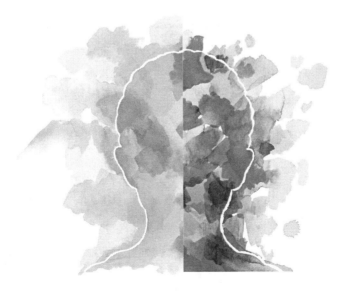

SEL Spotlight: Ernesto Durán
Regional Lead, CDE
Expanded Learning Division

As a young kid growing up in Mexico City—just my older brother and me, without parents—it was more important to learn survival skills than academic skills. Navigating our way through violence and danger without being robbed and beaten up or figuring out how to make a quick buck in order to eat was a bit more of a priority than memorizing the Pythagorean theorem. Hence, my view of SEL is through the lens of an immigrant, an English learner student, and a traumatized child.

Sadly, my experience is not as extreme or as rare as you might think. Many of the students we serve today have similar experiences, and most are not as fortunate as I am to have eventually landed in a safe environment, rich with opportunity and boundless options. On the contrary, in many of the neighborhoods in which we oversee after-school programs, kids are navigating through dangerous territory, encountering gangs, drug dealers, and prostitutes on their way to and from school. Is it any wonder they are not ready to learn when they arrive at school? I know I sure wasn't.

Neuroscience research is an ever-evolving field of study with new discoveries and the dispelling of old beliefs occurring by the minute. Emerging research on whether emotions are hard-wired versus learned is mixed. Currently, much attention is being given to both individual and cultural variances in how emotions are expressed and perceived. In other words, although there are some universal commonalities, the ways in which we perceive, express, and manage emotions vary from person to person as well as across various cultures. Previous studies established that the six hard-wired emotions are universal across all cultures. However, emerging research argues that even these basic emotions are subject to cultural influences and are shaped by one's individual life experiences.

Psychologist and neuroscientist Lisa Feldman Barrett (2017) explains this concept in terms we can all relate to, such as watching a crime report on television and making an immediate judgment as to whether the person in question is guilty or innocent based on how they behave and communicate. However, research tells us this snap judgment is actually based on our own individual and cultural perceptions of appropriate emotional expressions in a given situation. This emerging discovery that potentially none of our emotions are hard-wired and that instead they are all learned further supports the theory that SEL can and should be taught. Moreover, many experts like Barrett believe teaching children to recognize and manage their emotions in constructive ways supports both psychological development and academic growth.

Based on what we now know about the importance of the whole-child approach to education in ensuring successful transitions into college, career, and adulthood, exactly *when* in the K–12 system should this emphasis on SEL begin to take shape?

I had a student who came into first grade saying the meanest things about herself. She said she was stupid and couldn't read. She was quick to give up and just not try. It took the whole two years I had with her to break down that fixed negative mindset and build her confidence. I actually set up interventions to have her tell me five things she liked about herself every day and to end the day by telling me something that made her proud of herself. Before we could even make a dent in her academics, we had to address her self-image. This is how we address teaching in a holistic way. We have to take all aspects of a child's experience into consideration as we educate them.

All I Really Need to Know, I Learned in Kindergarten

Robert Fulghum's 1986 book *All I Really Need to Know, I Learned in Kindergarten* was a must read at the time of its release. In it, Fulghum cites his list of what we now know as SEL skills, typically acquired in kindergarten. Among them are: share everything, play fair, don't hit people, and say you're sorry when you hurt somebody. A fascinating study published in the *American Journal of Public Health* proves Fulghum was actually onto something. Following a group of kindergartners into adulthood, researchers found that mastery of SEL skills in early childhood is a stronger indicator of positive adult outcomes than are academic benchmarks. The findings indicated "statistically significant associations between measured social-emotional skills in kindergarten and key young adult outcomes across multiple domains of education, employment, criminal activity, substance abuse, and mental health" (Jones, Greenberg, and Crowley 2015). In other words, how very young children learn to interact socially with their peers, as well as how they learn to manage their own emotions, can more reliably predict how well they will fare in virtually all aspects of adult life—more so than grades, test scores, and GPAs.

That being said, the notion that students who reach middle school or high school without a solid SEL foundation are essentially "lost causes" is, in my opinion, rubbish. I have actually heard some educators say, "It's too late for them." Nonsense. Although early childhood is a prime time to establish these foundational skills, neuroscience research tells us that a second window of opportunity exists during adolescence, another critical point of *neuroplasticity* or *brain plasticity*—a developmental period when the human brain is most flexible in its ability to modify its connections or re-wire itself in order to cement certain foundational skills and behaviors.

In fact, some experts argue adolescence is an even more critical time for SEL than early childhood. "Within the field of positive psychology, interest is growing in how schools can facilitate adolescents' emotional growth, including the development of stronger self-control" (Steinberg 2015, 28). Steinberg explains how emotional development, particularly self-control and self-regulation, becomes increasingly challenging and critical to academic success as students progress through the grade levels. He argues that in the lower elementary grades, SEL skills such as perseverance tend not to be as much of an issue as they become in secondary education (2015). In other words,

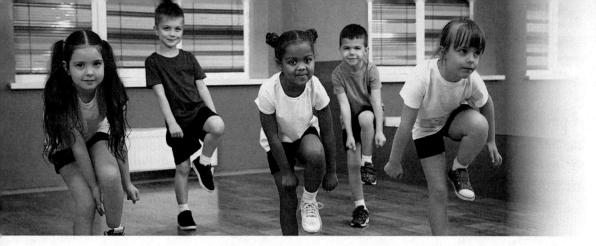

Steinberg contends that an intentional focus on developing students' SEL skills becomes even more critical to student success at the high school level where academic rigor increases and the stakes are higher. Furthermore, Steinberg connects the concepts of self-control and perseverance, stressing the increased importance of students resisting risky behaviors and persevering through to graduation day with what Duckworth would call "exhibiting grit." Recognition of adolescence being a vital second window of opportunity for SEL skill development may be partially responsible for the emerging support of SEL as a necessary counterbalance to a myopic focus on academic achievement as the sole indicator of student success in secondary education.

What's in a Name? Defining SEL Pedagogy

One of the potholes in paving the road to SEL implementation is in developing a common language and understanding of exactly what SEL is, which has proven quite challenging. Past incarnations of SEL include whole-child education, character education, positive youth development, and soft skills or noncognitive skills, just to name a few. Noncognitive skills can be defined as factors outside of "content knowledge and academic skills" (Farrington, as cited in Zinshteyn 2015, para. 4). In order to move support for SEL forward, it is essential that we strive toward a shared definition of SEL. For the purposes of this book, I use the definition of SEL provided by the Collaborative for Academic, Social, and Emotional Learning (CASEL). CASEL is considered the leading authority on all aspects of SEL and its application in K–12 education (Elias and Arnold 2006). CASEL defines SEL as:

> "The process through which children and adults acquire and effectively apply the knowledge, attitudes, and skills necessary to understand and manage emotions, set and achieve positive goals, feel and show empathy for others, establish and maintain positive relationships, and make responsible decisions" (CASEL n.d.).

CASEL originated in 1994 as a group of volunteer researchers and educators (Daniel Goleman among them) with the mission of establishing SEL as an essential part of the core K–12 education system. This organized effort around SEL grew to include the gathering and dissemination of evidence-based SEL practices and vetted curriculum, which, early on in the SEL movement, centered primarily on behavior modification and prevention programs rather than on a universal recognition of the need for SEL for all students. Although this early interest in youth education beyond academics was seen as encouraging, the problem that arose was the lack of knowledge educators needed to make informed decisions around adopting SEL curricula and practices. Recognizing this, CASEL's mission evolved to further the research and establish and recommend evidence-based practices for SEL for all students. Through collaborations with both the public and private sectors, CASEL was able to establish itself as a vehicle for promoting SEL as a "framework that addresses the needs of young people and helps to align and coordinate school programs and programming" (CASEL n.d.). CASEL has established five interrelated core competencies essential to the development of SEL skills: self-awareness, self-management, social awareness, relationship skills, and responsible decision-making (figure 1.1).

Figure 1.1

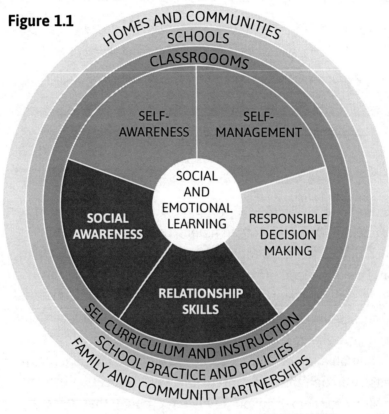

©CASEL 2017

Few would argue against the value of instilling these types of skills in students. However, the methods and strategies implemented to cultivate such skills have become the subject of much debate. These are areas we will continue to explore in subsequent chapters throughout the book. Today, CASEL continues to light the path for the development and promotion of all things SEL, providing educators with detailed frameworks from which to build SEL infrastructures and abundant tools and resources to draw from in creating SEL toolkits. There is much to explore on the CASEL website at **www.casel.org**.

Why the Push for SEL Now?

Despite the extensive school reform initiatives K–12 education has experienced over the past several decades, we have failed to significantly move the needle on the academic performance of U.S. students. According to the National Assessment of Education Progress (NAEP), reading and math scores among U.S. teens have remained static over the past 40 years (Steinberg 2015). America's abysmal standing on the global K–12 stage is well-documented, which begs the question: What are we missing?

Considering that current research cites the importance of nonacademic skill development in supporting overall student success, how do American students fare in the SEL arena? U.S. high school students "lag behind many of their international counterparts in an important skill—self-control" (Steinberg 2015, 30). Self-control, also known as self-regulation, can be identified as the ability to manage emotions and to delay gratification, which is a prime indicator for future success in adulthood.

You may be familiar with Walter Mischel's famous marshmallow experiment, which took place from the 1960s through the 1980s. From this landmark study, we learned how a child's ability to delay gratification (exhibit self-control or self-regulation) from eating a marshmallow seemed to directly correlate with their future success. The study revealed that the longer a child's "wait time" in succumbing to the temptation of eating a marshmallow, the greater their academic success in later years (Duckworth 2016; Tough 2012). More recently, building on the marshmallow study, Duckworth discovered that in order for kids to delay gratification, they had to be *intrinsically motivated* to do so; if a child doesn't like marshmallows in the first place, then Mischel's marshmallow experiment is not much of a test of willpower. Additionally, it is important to note that if a child comes to school hungry, they may not be able to delay the gratification of the offered food.

How does this translate to academics? Students must find value and engagement in the learning process and objectives in order to feel motivated to achieve. They also need to feel a sense of belonging and connectedness to the learning environment. There is consensus that the types of SEL characteristics needed to persevere, delay gratification, and engage in learning are malleable traits that can be taught and cultivated (Duckworth 2016; Tough 2012). These findings support what many educators have known intuitively for some time:

> "Teachers across the country explained that SEL increases student interest in learning, improves student behavior, prevents and reduces bullying, and improves school climate. In all, more than three quarters of teachers believe a larger focus on SEL will be a major benefit to students" (Bridgeland and Bruce 2013).

With substantial support for SEL now established, how do we begin to move from embracing the importance of SEL skill development to implementing SEL practices?

State Standards for K–12 SEL

As any educator who has been in the field for any length of time can attest, what gets measured or mandated gets taught or funded. In the case of SEL, mandating and measuring these types of skills is the subject of debate, which we will explore further in subsequent chapters. The controversy over whether states should mandate SEL standards may be the rationale behind some states opting to support social and emotional learning in ways other than mandated standards. Largely as a result of CASEL's work, Illinois (where CASEL is based) was among the first states to adopt mandated K–12 SEL standards. Figure 1.2 illustrates how, as of September 2018, 14 states have followed suit and issued standards for SEL in K–12 schools, and all 50 states now have SEL standards for preschool (CASEL 2018).

Figure 1.2 State SEL Statistics

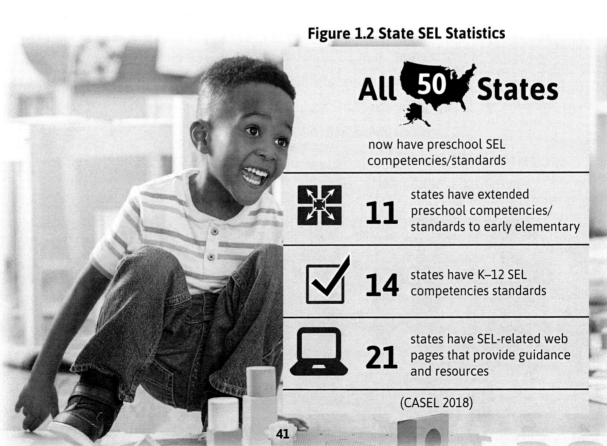

All **50** States

now have preschool SEL competencies/standards

11 states have extended preschool competencies/ standards to early elementary

14 states have K–12 SEL competencies standards

21 states have SEL-related web pages that provide guidance and resources

(CASEL 2018)

Summary

In recent years, the K–12 system has put a myopic focus on academics and standardized testing. Yet, despite these concentrated efforts through myriad education reform initiatives, we have failed to significantly move the needle on student achievement. American students still lag far behind many of their international peers. So, what are we missing?

A robust body of evidence is now able to answer that question. And the answer is SEL. Thanks in large part to the 2015 Every Student Succeeds Act (ESSA) citing "nonacademic" indicators as a factor in measuring student success, we are now seeing nationwide support for the implementation of SEL in K–12 education. Although the evidence and support are there, the question educators and policy makers are now grappling with is *What exactly is SEL, and how do we teach it?* Using CASEL's definition and framework, we will continue exploring this question in the coming chapters.

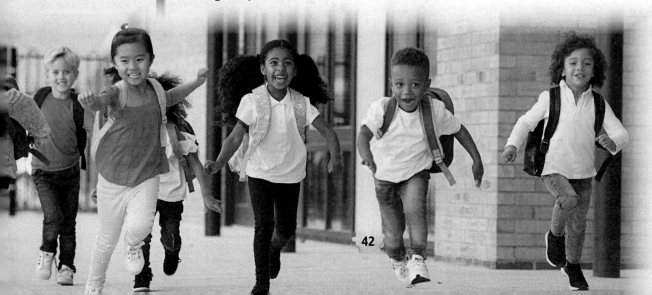

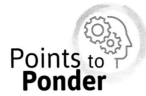

Points to Ponder

1. Reflect on your initial responses to these statements. How have your responses changed?

   » SEL is a fairly new concept in education.

   » SEL and academics are two unrelated skill sets.

   » SEL is meant only for very young children.

Points to **Ponder** (cont.)

2. Do you feel you have a better grasp on what SEL is? What questions remain?

3. Where is your state, county, district, or program in terms of support for SEL? (Visit the State Scan Scorecard on the CASEL website for the most current information: **casel.org/state-scan-scorecard-project-2**.)

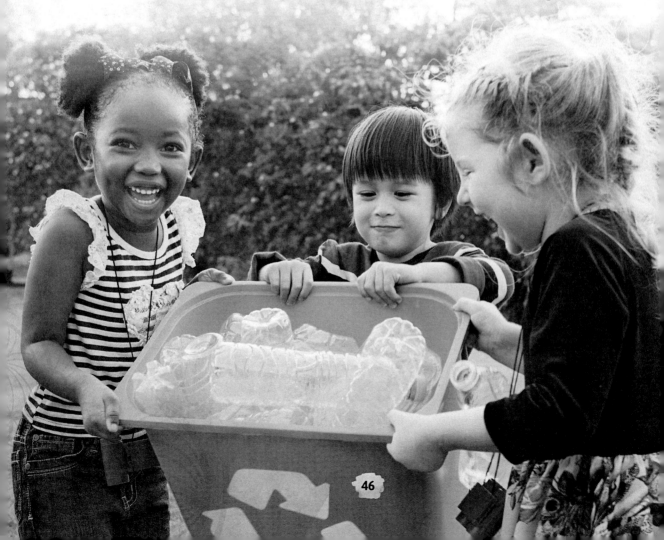

The time has come for an Emotion Revolution in our nation's education system. Research shows that emotions drive learning, decision-making, relationships, and mental health. Evidence-based approaches to social and emotional learning lead to higher academic performance, greater teacher effectiveness, and enhanced school climate.

—Marc Brackett, Ph.D., Founding Director
Yale Center for Emotional Intelligence

Chapter Two

The Impact of SEL on Education and Society

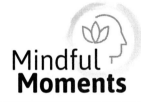

Mindful Moments

* Before reading this chapter, take a moment to think about SEL from a broader perspective. What impact do you think having comprehensive SEL practices integrated in all aspects of the K–12 educational system might have on the following issues in education today?

    » school climate and safety

    » opportunity/achievement gap

    » chronic absenteeism

    » graduation rates

* How do you imagine a greater emphasis on SEL might manifest itself in society as a whole, both locally and globally?

This emotion revolution in education is taking hold not only in the United States but around the world. A recent body of research from the Organization for Economic Co-operation and Development (OECD) included a longitudinal analysis across nine countries and "found that a number of socio-emotional skills including self-esteem, self-efficacy, and sociability consistently played a particularly important role in certain cultures. . . . There is also a common set of skills that seem to matter wherever you are" (Miyamoto 2015). Although there is bound to be some variation across cultures as to how people perceive and express emotions, the common thread is that emotions play an important role, regardless of your location on the globe.

Something unique to the field of education (as compared to other professions or industries) is the fact that our customer and our product are one and the same—our students. They are both who we serve and what we create and send forth into society. It's our enormously important responsibility as educators to produce quality products. So, how can we best prepare our students for life beyond school?

What's Your Why?

Start with *why*. Author and motivational speaker Simon Sinek is credited with this concept, which is now being applied in both the public and private sectors. Ask yourself *why* you do what you do. As an educator, I have always felt that the ultimate goal of educating students should be to prepare them for a successful adult life, which in large part includes the workforce. If one's education does not prepare one for a successful adulthood, then frankly, what good is it? That said, in addition to academics, what skills do students *really* need in order to achieve success beyond school?

Twenty-First-Century Skills and College and Career Readiness

"Research suggests that there are 25 social and emotional competencies that are most often linked to [workplace] success" (Goleman 1998, as cited by Elias and Arnold 2006, 59–60). These 25 SEL workplace competencies are presented under five headings: self-awareness, self-regulation, motivation, social awareness, and social skills—a striking alignment with CASEL's five core competencies for SEL education. As Daniel Goleman explains, "Four of five companies are trying to promote emotional intelligence in their employees. Although American employers clearly are willing to help their workers become more socially and emotionally competent, they would prefer to have the schools do it before those employees grow up and go to work. And for good reason: It is easier to learn these skills when one is young" (Elias and Arnold 2006, 59). Although certain academic skills are essential to most careers, employers overwhelmingly cite SEL skills as what is most needed, and most lacking, in the current employee pool (Dowd and Liedtka 1994, as cited by Elias and Arnold 2006).

SEL skills such as these were noted by employers as being far more important than IQ and technical skills in determining employee success. Even in highly technical fields, most employees will eventually reach a "threshold," at which point colleagues essentially become equals in terms of technical skill. However, it is the individual's competency in the realm of social and emotional

> The three skills employers cited as most desirable were interpersonal skills, communication skills, and initiative (Dowd and Liedtka 1994, as cited by Elias and Arnold 2006).

skills that will set them apart from coworkers lacking such skills. SEL skills developed in childhood and adolescence transfer to become workplace skills such as teamwork, communication, and collaboration (Elias and Arnold 2006).

Moreover, a Penn State University policy brief on the long-term economic impact of improving childhood SEL skills states that "the benefits of investing in social emotional health are increasingly evident. . . . A growing base of research examining the value of implementing SEL skill-building interventions . . . found over an $11 return on investment for each dollar invested" (Jones, Crowley, and Greenberg 2017, 2). This discovery has led to interest and support of SEL extending beyond educators to economists and governmental policy makers. SEL skills "increase the likelihood of success in the workplace. . . . Becoming more apparent is their potential influence on, and relevance to, economic outcomes" (2017, 4). The study explains that disadvantaged students in underserved communities are likely to experience the greatest impact with regard to SEL benefits and outcomes. This supports the contention that SEL can be a means of narrowing the opportunity gap that exists between students on each end of the socioeconomic spectrum and leads to the academic divide known as the *achievement gap.*

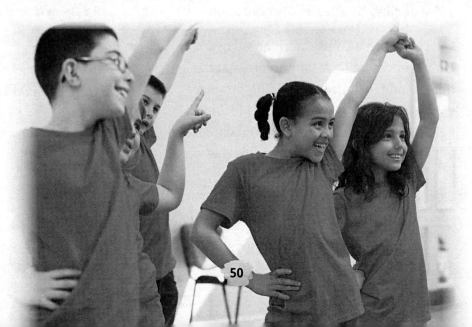

Addressing Equity: Mitigating the Opportunity Gap

The achievement gap is a term educators and researchers use to identify the significant divide that exists in academic performance levels between high- and low-performing students, as evidenced by standardized testing. Typically, this great divide falls clearly along socioeconomic and racial lines, with low-performing students of color, English Learners (ELs), and high-poverty populations performing far below their wealthier, white counterparts (Tough 2012).

"A curious transformation in the political landscape surrounding education and poverty in America has transpired in recent decades. What were once two separate and distinct issues—poverty and education—have merged into one, and it's about the achievement gap between rich and poor—the very real fact that overall, children who grow up in poor families in the United States are doing very badly in school" (Tough 2012, 187).

In other words, we now know that socioeconomic status and academic achievement are inextricably intertwined and correlated. Given an understanding of the effect poverty has on student success, what steps can we take to counteract these effects and mitigate the achievement gap? First, let's examine the term *achievement gap.*

Two problems exist with the term achievement gap. First, it ranks students based solely on their academic skills, as evidenced by standardized testing. In so doing, it discounts *nonacademic* skills, such as SEL competencies. Secondly, "Research has shown that lower-income students have far less access to learning and enrichment opportunities than do their wealthier peers" (Davis 2015, 2).

Findings such as these have led many in education to the acknowledgement of a predicating *opportunity gap* contributing to the academic achievement gap. After-school enrichment and expanded learning programs are one way to address the opportunity gap by exposing students to *enrichment* opportunities, similar to those experienced by their wealthier peers, mitigating the effects of poverty and helping to close the achievement gap. For instance, students being picked up after school to participate in music and art classes or team sports have a marked advantage over their less-affluent peers in accessing experiences that foster the development of SEL skills. Structured after-school programs aim to bridge this divide and create equitable access to enrichment activities as well as provide additional academic support in an effort to create a level playing field for all students.

Enriching Learning Opportunities for All Students

One primary example of an enrichment opportunity is the school field trip. Unlike their more affluent counterparts, students from lower socioeconomic backgrounds often lack exposure to enriching experiences, such as family excursions to distant locales, museums, historical landmarks, or other educational experiences outside the classroom. In speaking with students and staff from some of our after-school programs, the benefit of such enrichment experiences is clearly evident.

Sally, a high school teacher who works with students on both ends of the socioeconomic spectrum, shared a recent field trip experience. She took 21 teenagers on an overnight trip to a city just three hours away for a student leadership council. Jared-James, a 19-year-old senior who participated in the trip, shared his impressions with me:

"Well first we went to this Hall of Justice thing. They talk about how the court works, what they do—they give a motivational speech. Then we did a scavenger hunt around the old town, just looking at the old places and learning some stuff."

Of greater interest to him during this field trip was his exposure to new experiences and locales. He expressed enthusiasm about the environment and people he observed, saying:

"The city was like New York, but with less people. People with business suits, nice cars. I was like, Dang, I want to be like them—walk around in a business suit like that—my nice car—be like, I worked hard for this, you know?"

In comparing his level of enthusiasm for the educational intention of the trip with his enthusiasm about exposure to a new environment, which do you think he will remember? What made the greatest impact on him: the academic experience or the social and emotional experience? This is not to say we shouldn't focus on the academic benefits of such excursions but rather that we be cognizant, and even intentional, as to the social and emotional benefits and learning that come from such experiences.

Societal Climate Affects School Climate

Recently, a colleague shared with me that many students in her districts had started coming to school with two backpacks. When staff investigated why this was occurring in significant numbers, they were taken aback by what they uncovered. Students and their parents reluctantly revealed that in light of the current political climate, particularly in regard to immigration reform issues, many undocumented families had begun to take precautions should the time come when their children might arrive home from school to find their parents had been deported or detained by authorities. Hence, one backpack was for books and school supplies, and the other was for clothing and toiletries should the need arise to spend the night (or who knows how long) somewhere other than home.

There is no shortage of news on the turbulent environment in which we all reside. The state of California, for instance, is home to the largest population of undocumented immigrants in the nation, with 250,000 of them being students. "Immigrant students are one of the most vulnerable populations served in public education. . . . Research shows the changes in policies have negatively impacted immigrant students. . . . New studies reveal a discernable decline in academic performance, school attendance, [and] enrollment in school-based programs and children's health services" (O'Neil 2018).

Regardless of where you sit on the political spectrum, as an educator concerned with the well-being of all of your students, you can appreciate the enormous level of stress and fear this scenario brings to many in our communities. That stress impacts a child's ability to learn and achieve as well as the overall school climate (O'Neil 2018). This is just one of many examples illustrating the turbulent culture our students are exposed to daily. SEL is needed now more than ever.

SEL Spotlight: Kris Hinrichsen
Teacher, Chinook Open Optional Program

Communicating with parents is very valuable for SEL work. I communicate to parents what lessons we have learned in the week, what skills we are practicing, and any new language their kids might come home with. I got some great feedback after a lesson on prejudice and discrimination when a family went to see a movie about a girl who wasn't being treated fairly because she was a girl, and the child walked out telling the parents that the girl was discriminated against and that wasn't right. My heart leapt with joy for a six-year-old to take that lesson and apply it to the outside world so quickly.

The Big Picture on School Climate, Safety, and Mental Health

Speaking with Dr. Jennifer Freed and her colleague Rendy Freeman, whose work with SEL programming for teens is featured in *Preparing Youth to Thrive: Promising Practices for Social & Emotional Learning* (Smith et al. 2016), provided a big picture perspective on the need for SEL in creating a safe and healthy school climate. Both are licensed therapists and cofounders of the nonprofit organization AHA!, which stands for Attitude, Harmony, and Achievement. AHA! was born out of the tragedy of the Columbine school shooting in 1999. This event served as a wake-up call for the two who identified, through decades of counseling teens, that the Columbine event was symbolic of a more pervasive national epidemic of unhappy, ill-adjusted "lost souls in schools" struggling to survive in educational environments that are not meeting their social and emotional needs. Dr. Freed explained, "We wanted to create a program where teens specifically felt like there was a place where they could be themselves and belong." The pair knew that SEL was a must-have for all adolescents; however, they soon identified that it was of particular need for at-risk students. "We went into continuation schools with our SEL program and immediately saw that attendance went up. Their test scores went up, and the academics [school-wide averages] went up in a school that was really struggling" (Smith et al. 2016). Along with mental health professionals such as these, the education community, legislators, and policy makers have now come together to acknowledge the broad impact of SEL.

Legislation on SEL

Federal Legislation

The CASEL website is an excellent resource for keeping abreast of current legislation on SEL policy. Listed on the following page is the latest on pending legislation, along with some background on early legislation that laid the foundation for SEL policy today.

Among SEL's strongest policy champions is Congressman Tim Ryan of Ohio. Ryan's latest proposals for SEL includes the Chronic Absenteeism Reduction Act of 2017 to amend the Elementary and Secondary Education Act (ESEA) and allow local educational agencies to use federal funds for programs and activities that address chronic absenteeism. Chronic absenteeism is defined as students missing 10 percent or more of the school year. The bill is primarily built around implementing mentorship programs as a bridge between home and school to encourage regular attendance as well as a way of "providing personnel training to build positive school climates and promote social-emotional learning" (CASEL n.d.). Also introduced by Ryan in 2017 was the Teacher Health and Wellness Act. "This bill directs the National Institutes of Health to carry out a five-year study on reducing teacher stress and increasing teacher retention and well-being by implementing and analyzing the results of any of several types of innovative approaches that include:

- → workplace wellness programs;
- → social emotional learning programs;
- → teacher stress management programs;
- → mentoring and induction programs during the school year and teacher pre-service;
- → organizational interventions such as principal training programs;
- → teacher residency programs;
- → complementary health approaches, such as mindfulness meditation; and
- → school reorganization" (CASEL, n.d.).

Early on in the SEL movement, most of the proposed legislation centered on teacher training and professional development. This focus is in alignment with the data gleaned from educators and administrators as to the lack of understanding, expertise, and confidence in teaching SEL. Some of the early proposals that propelled us to where we are today are outlined below.

In 2015, Tim Ryan introduced the Academic, Social, and Emotional Learning Act (H.R. 850). This bill uses CASEL's definition and core competencies of SEL to guide programming and allows for funding of educator professional development of SEL practices through the amendment of the Elementary and Secondary Education Act (ESEA) (CASEL n.d.).

Additional legislation known as the Supporting Social and Emotional Learning Act (H.R. 497) was introduced by California Representative Susan Davis in 2015. This bill proposed to "require highly qualified teachers to have preparation in the understanding, use, and development of social and emotional learning programming" (CASEL n.d.). The language in this bill unequivocally describes how the U.S. educational system has failed to impart equal emphasis on both academic and nonacademic skills and advocates that "social and emotional learning should be included as a central component of our education system. Federal law needs to include language that prioritizes social and emotional learning for educators" (H.R. 497 2016, para. 10).

The Collaborating States Initiative (CSI)

Perhaps the most significant of all SEL legislation is the Collaborating States Initiative, known as CSI. The following description of the CSI is located on the CASEL website:

The CSI materials and resources mentioned in the description can be accessed from the CASEL website. CASEL also provides guidance on selecting evidenced-based SEL curriculum, which it has fully evaluated.

Should SEL Be Mandated?

The momentum of the SEL movement is building, evidenced by the number of states jumping on board by issuing SEL standards and exerting other types of influence and guidance in support of SEL integration. This is encouraging to see as a champion of SEL. However, there are those who believe the trend toward mandating SEL and its potential use as a factor in schoolwide

"CASEL's Collaborating States Initiative (CSI), launched in 2016, works with states and school districts to help develop goals, guidelines, programs, and plans that will help them promote social and emotional learning (SEL) statewide. Over time the participating state education leaders have developed a wide variety of materials and resources to promote SEL in their states. Sharing resources and building a nationwide learning community of state educational leaders is central to the CSI" (CASEL n.d.).

accountability systems are cause for concern. For some, the mere idea of measuring something that many consider to be individual "character traits" flies in the face of what this movement away from standardized testing is all about. For many, the move toward measuring SEL is, at best, highly subjective and, at worst, outright offensive.

Researcher Angela Duckworth, albeit a strong supporter of SEL, has been among the most outspoken critics of using SEL measures as a school accountability indicator, forcefully asserting that it should not be done and that it is a "bad idea" (Zernike 2016). Duckworth's argument is motivated by the nascent nature of SEL research and her belief that attaching any high-stakes accountability measures just yet would be premature (Duckworth 2016).

From a global standpoint, there are others who agree with Duckworth's argument, particularly in terms of developing a measurement tool that is valid across all student populations. "The evidence base useful for teachers and parents to raise children's socio-emotional skills is still very limited. This is due, in part, to the under-developed measurement instruments available for measuring socio-emotional skills across countries, cultures, and population groups" (Miyamoto 2015). In brief, the jury is still out on whether or not SEL should be mandated, and the pros and cons of using SEL as an accountability measure are still being weighed. However, based on the abundant research in support of SEL, deciding whether to use it as an accountability metric should not deter or hinder our efforts to implement SEL moving forward. Remember your "why."

Are You Ready to Assess?

According to the American Institutes for Research (AIR), "assessing individuals' social and emotional (SE) knowledge, attitudes, and skills is a complex task. It requires careful consideration of the assessment purpose, rigor, practicality, burden, and ethics. Once you have considered these factors and have determined that you are, in fact, ready to assess, you are ready to act and choose an assessment tool to achieve your desired outcome" (SEL Solutions 2015). The AIR website is another great resource for SEL assessment tools, broken down by grade levels, educational settings, format of the tool, and the specific SEL skills to be measured. Also available from AIR is a planning tool that focuses on the integration of SEL in both the regular school day and the after-school program. Visit the AIR website at **www.air.org**.

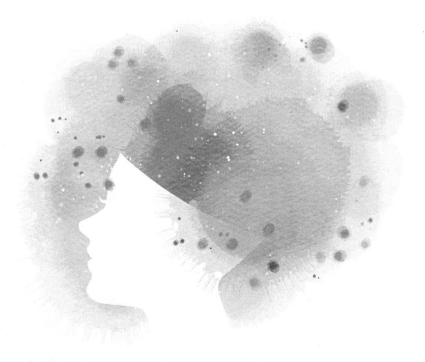

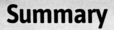

Summary

SEL should be viewed in terms of its impact on the overarching, universal priorities for education as a whole or, in other words, the big picture. SEL is not an isolated practice suitable only for certain environments or select student populations. All students and all schools need SEL to cultivate safe, healthy, and effective learning environments for students of all ages and backgrounds.

K–12 educators across the nation largely agree SEL skills would positively impact workforce readiness (87 percent), school attendance and graduation (80 percent), life success (87 percent), college preparation (78 percent), and academic success (75 percent) (Bridgeland, Bruce, and Hariharan 2013, 17). As we begin to accept that SEL is not a "nice-to-have" but a "must-have" for all students in all educational settings, the next step in the process is *creating environments* conducive to fostering SEL skill development, which we will explore in depth in the next chapter.

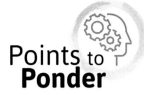

Points to Ponder

1. After reading this chapter, how has your perspective on the big picture of SEL changed? What impact do you think comprehensive SEL practices being integrated in all aspects of the K–12 educational system might have on the following?

» school climate and safety

» opportunity/achievement gap

Points to **Ponder** *(cont.)*

» chronic absenteeism

» graduation rates

2. How do you imagine a greater emphasis on SEL in education will manifest itself in society as a whole, both locally and globally?

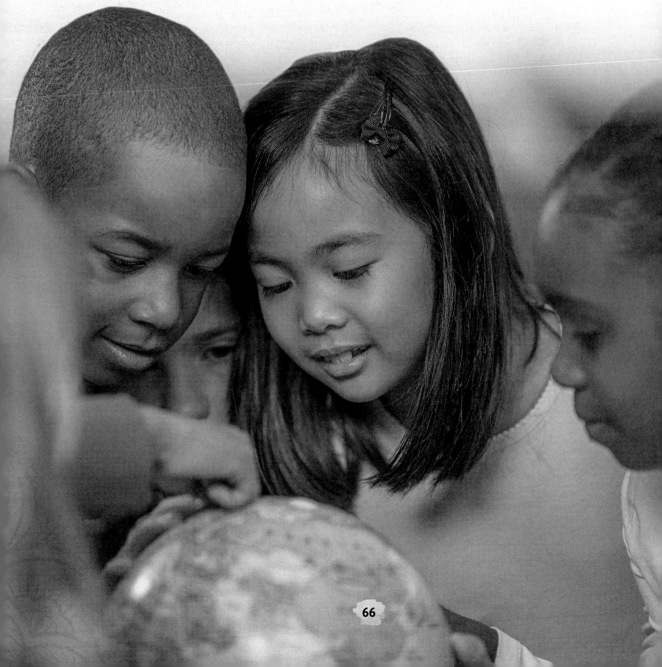

If we want to improve a child's grit or self-control, what we need to change first is his environment.

—Paul Tough

Chapter Three

Creating
SEL Environments

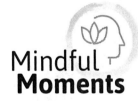

Mindful Moments

* How do you envision an SEL environment? What would it look like?

* Consider the differences between these two statements:

    » Educators should prioritize social and emotional learning.

    » Educators should recognize that learning is social and emotional.

Any time an educator wants to try something new in the classroom, one of the first things that comes to mind is *when? When am I going to fit this into my class, program, curriculum, or day?*

The best response I have heard to this argument came from an Illinois school district leader, Gene Olsen. He said, "SEL is not one more thing on the plate. It is the plate!" (CASEL 2018, 20).

In other words, as we know from Maslow's Hierarchy of Needs, we must first have our basic needs met before we can aspire to higher-level goals (McLeod n.d.). Along with food, shelter, and safety, social and emotional needs are essential to a healthy environment for all human beings. Maslow's model stresses the importance of individuals, children, and adults alike having a sense of belonging, love, and self-esteem. Students need a solid social and emotional foundation before they can effectively learn and achieve. In fact, educators are starting to use the phrase "Maslow before Bloom," referring to Bloom's taxonomy of educational objectives, which most educators are familiar with (figure 3.1).

Figure 3.1 Maslow's Hierarchy and Bloom's Taxonomy

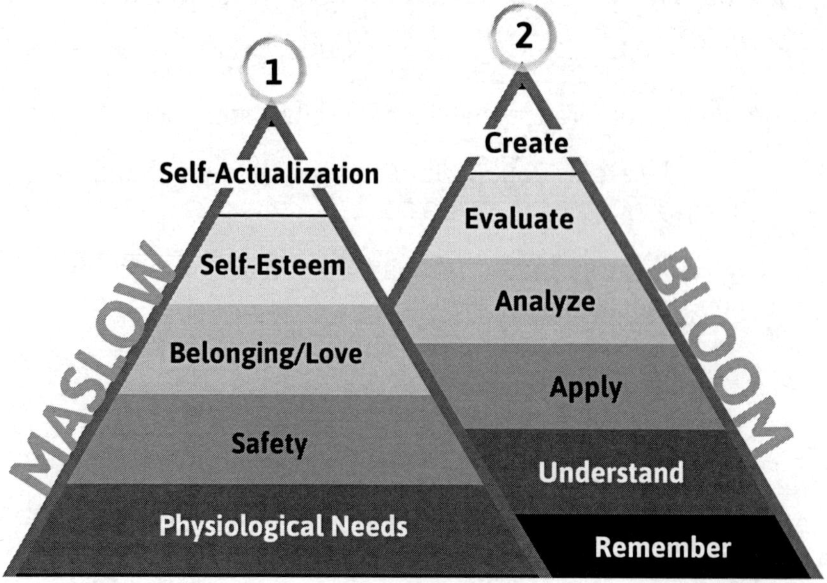

Ensuring Students' Safety

Although the recent emphasis on SEL is a welcome change in education, in the rush to jump on the SEL bandwagon with practices such as mindfulness, what is sometimes overlooked is the most fundamental of all social and emotional needs: safety—physical and emotional. Educators and parents alike struggle with how to *teach* kids to be safe, both in the real world and online. While there is no shortage of "child safety" resources, the implementation of specific prevention programming and the knowledge and training needed to teach such curriculum is lacking. Educators are well aware of our status as mandated reporters of child abuse and neglect. However, most are not familiar with the signs and statistics surrounding child sex trafficking and exploitation or the available resources to educate and empower students in the fight to prevent victimization. Many educators may be stunned to learn that one in ten children will be sexually abused before their eighteenth birthday and one in seven children reported as runaways were likely victims of child sex trafficking (NCMEC 2018, 2019).

The National Center for Missing and Exploited Children (NCMEC) is the leading authority on Child Safety and Prevention Education. NCMEC deals with all aspects of child endangerment, including sexual abuse, child abduction, and human trafficking. These are difficult topics to discuss or even think about, and they are topics we tend to avoid. However, if our students are not safe from harm (both physical and emotional), how can they even begin to learn and achieve? As uncomfortable as it might be, we must face these issues head-on.

As educators and mandated reporters, turning a blind eye and pretending these issues don't exist is not an option for us. So how can we be proactive in ensuring the safety of our students both inside and outside the learning environment? We start by educating ourselves.

SEL Spotlight: Ernesto Durán
Regional Lead, CDE
Expanded Learning Division

I routinely ran away from school in Mexico City, beginning at seven years old. I was chronically absent and eventually expelled. My brother (and legal guardian) was told by school administration to "bring me back *when I was ready to learn*." That didn't happen until I was 11. Thanks to my 18-year-old brother, I learned to read, write, and do basic math at home. During those four years of home-schooling, I finally developed some sense of security and stability. My brother did his best to provide a safe and supportive home environment amidst the turmoil and chaos of our lives. Having his support, and having attained some basic academic skills, I found the confidence to return to school feeling prepared and emotionally stable.

How much do you know about these topics and how to educate students in a way that is age-appropriate and that will empower them to recognize and avoid such dangers, be it online or in the real world?

Based on their vast knowledge and expertise in this area, NCMEC has developed K–12 curricula known as KidSmartz and NetSmartz to educate and protect children and teens in both real-world and online scenarios. In pilots of the curriculum, students exhibited greater awareness and recognition of potentially dangerous situations. Feedback from staff indicates the lessons also informed adult knowledge as well as strengthened the staff's relationships with students as "trusted adults" in students' lives. Staff members have also reported that, despite the sensitive nature of the subject matter, the lessons are simple and easy to deliver. As much as we may want to shy away from this topic, it is a reality we must face in order to empower our students with the tools needed to protect themselves. Visit the NCMEC website (**www.missingkids.com**) to continue learning on this important issue.

Setting the Stage for SEL: Environmental Building Blocks

Ultimately, SEL practices and strategies should be integrated into all aspects of the learning environment—across all grade levels and content areas, and both within and outside of the traditional school day and classroom setting. That said, where do we begin to realize this vision for the future of SEL? Let's start by establishing a research-based framework for SEL implementation.

CASEL advocates for a four-pronged approach to SEL implementation (figure 3.2), which requires incorporating one or more of the following components:

Figure 3.2 CASEL's Approach to SEL Implementation

Free-standing lessons using the SAFE approach (see *instruction* framework on page 72)

Universal teaching practices incorporated schoolwide

Integration of SEL in academic content

Schoolwide SEL initiatives facilitated by all school staff, including non-teaching staff

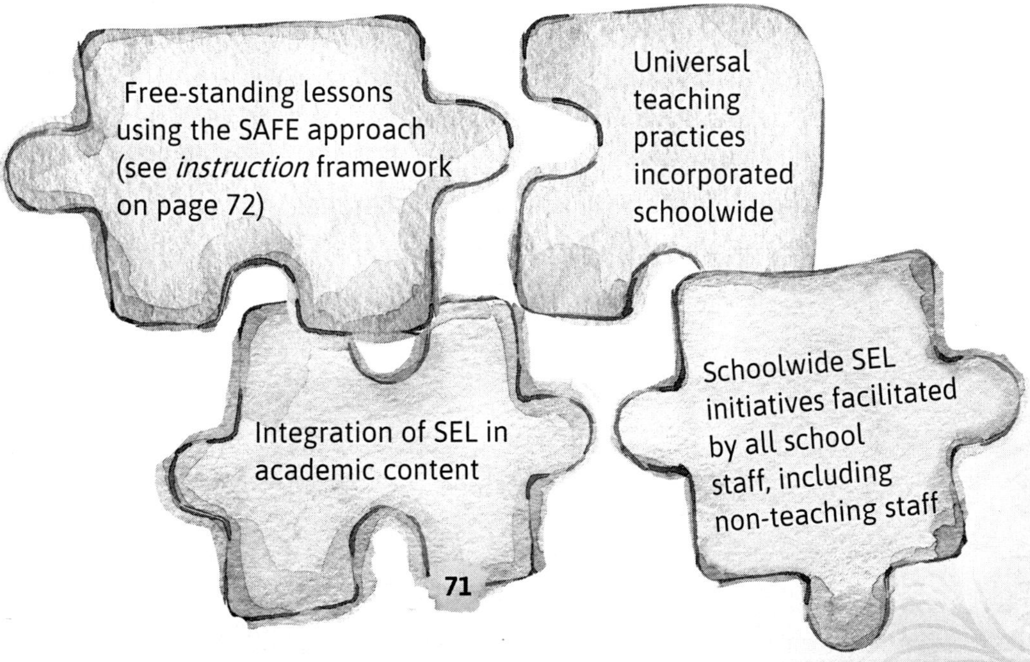

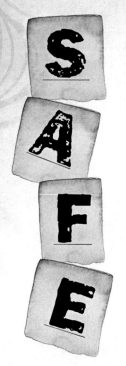

Similar to the implementation framework, CASEL also provides a framework for the effective delivery of SEL instruction, known as the "SAFE" approach. The acronym SAFE stands for:

Sequenced activities coordinated to cultivate SEL skill building

Active learning, such as project-based and hands-on learning to support mastery

Focused intentional emphasis on the cultivation of SEL

Explicit in the development of specific SEL skill sets

(CASEL 2015)

Ultimately, the vision for SEL is to implement and adopt these frameworks in their entirety throughout all of K–12 education. However, to get the SEL ball rolling in your school, program, or professional practice, CASEL recommends tackling just one or two of the implementation points to start.

In addition to CASEL's framework, the Aspen Institute has also released a very similar 3-pronged approach, essentially combining CASEL strategies 2 and 4 into one, which they refer to as *creating an environment* that fosters SEL skill development. The creation of that environment extends even to the hiring and training practices of teachers and staff, as well as using data from students, parents, and other stakeholders on issues such as school climate to guide thinking and inform planning of SEL practices. Aspen's recommendations were released in August 2018 in a report titled, *Realizing the Vision* for SEL in the K-12 setting. The Aspen Institute is another excellent SEL resource. For more information visit their website at **www.aspeninstitute.org**.

As we move from theory to practice, let's look at potential entry points for introducing SEL into our teaching and learning environments.

The Role of School Leadership in Creating SEL Environments

Principals, district administrators, and school site leaders play a pivotal role in creating an environment where SEL practices thrive. A recent national report entitled "Ready to Lead" surveyed over 800 Pre-K–12 public school principals, including interviews with a number of superintendents and input from district-level research and evaluation experts, to capture the leadership perspective and key insights around four major areas of SEL:

- ➡ **Attitudes about SEL:** Principals understand, value, and are committed to developing SEL skills.

- ➡ **SEL Implementation:** Support for SEL is high, but implementation varies greatly.

- ➡ **The Path to Increased SEL:** Principals want more SEL training for teachers and access to research-based strategies.

- ➡ **Assessing SEL:** Most principals believe SEL skills can be accurately measured and assessed (DePaoli, Atwell, and Bridgeland 2017, 3–5).

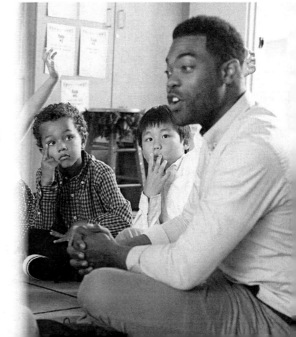

In concert with previous teacher surveys, principals overwhelmingly support incorporating SEL into their schools. "Nearly all principals (98 percent) believe students from all types of backgrounds—both affluent and poor—would benefit from learning social and emotional skills in schools" (DePaoli, Atwell, and Bridgeland 2017, 3–4). With such overwhelming support for SEL, why are only about one-third of principals implementing SEL on a school-wide level?

The report sheds light, from the school principal's perspective, on identifying circumstances that impact both successful SEL implementation and student outcomes:

- ➡ Principals value SEL but need greater knowledge and support to effectively implement schoolwide, evidence-based SEL programming.

- ➡ When superintendents and other district leaders are driving SEL and implementation is high, successful outcomes are much more likely.

- ➡ A lack of time and teacher training—in both pre-service education and in-school professional development—are critical barriers to implementing SEL.

- ➡ School and district leaders are open to having better data on students' social and emotional competencies to improve schoolwide SEL programming and student outcomes but need better training to do so (DePaoli, Atwell, and Bridgeland 2017, 41–42).

Many of these can be categorized as *external* factors, outside the purview of the school site leader. But let's look at a potential starting point that is within reach.

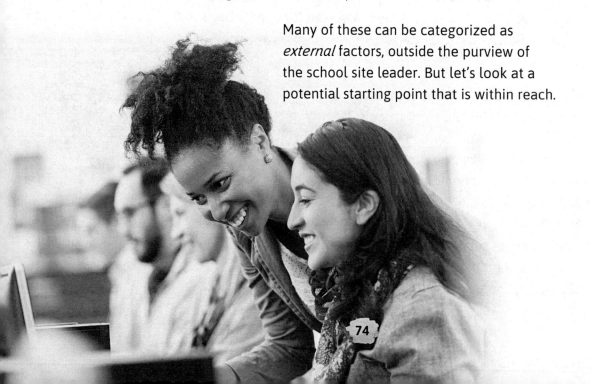

Happy Schools Need Happy Teachers

Emerging SEL research supports the importance of starting with adult practice. This means that we must first take stock of our own understanding and self-regulation of emotions before we can attempt to work with students on developing these types of skills. In "10 Ways We Made Our School Happier," Principal Tracey Smith writes:

> As educators, one of the biggest challenges we face is learning how to put our health and happiness first. My first thought was that I needed to put the students' well-being first, but I discovered that I needed to start with my staff instead (2018, para. 2).

Principal Smith is onto something. A study published in the *Journal of Positive Behavior Interventions* stated: "it's no secret that teaching is a stressful profession. However, when stress interferes with personal and emotional well-being at such a severe level, the relationships teachers have with students are likely to suffer, much like any relationship would in a high stress environment" (Herman, Hickmon-Rosa, and Reinke 2017). This scenario can be summed up by the title of a book written by Neila A. Connors: *If You Don't Feed the Teachers, They Eat the Students!*

Any one of us who has spent time working with children and teens doesn't need a study to know that educating youth, while extremely rewarding, can be very stressful. We may not realize how we pass that stress along to our students and how it impacts their behavior and academic achievement. According to the aforementioned study, 93 percent of teachers report "high levels of job-related stress." And "classrooms with highly stressed teachers usually have the poorest student outcomes, including lower grades and frequent behavior problems" (Herman, Hickmon-Rosa, and Reinke 2017). Additionally, stressed-out teachers lead to burned-out teachers, which lead to challenges with teacher retention. It's a vicious cycle in our profession. Included in the study are recommendations for mitigating high-stress educational settings:

"Building initiatives and programs that promote mental health practices and overall health can be extremely beneficial for teachers. We as a society need to consider methods that create nurturing school environments not just for students, but for the adults who work there" (Herman, Hickmon-Rosa, and Reinke 2017).

Although it is no surprise to most of us that teaching is stressful, it raises a deeper question—what practices can we implement to deescalate our stress levels?

Practice Mindful Moments

Meditation, an age-old practice recently gaining in popularity, might be a strategy you already use in your personal life, but it can also be applied professionally. There are many different approaches to the practice of meditation. The beauty is in the simplicity. Unlike some of the fad exercise programs we have all fallen for from time to time, meditation requires no bulky apparatus we have to find a place to store when not in use. That said, today there are high-tech approaches to meditation as well. Headspace, which brands itself as "a gym membership for your mind," is accessible from an app on your mobile device. It is quick, simple, and easy to include as a daily routine that is rooted in mindfulness. Headspace is currently rolling out a campaign to provide educators and students with access to their meditation applications. Additionally, they are in the process of developing curriculum for K–12 learning environments to guide teachers in implementing meditation and mindfulness practices for specific SEL-related skill development. For more information on bringing Headspace to your learning environment, visit their website at **www.headspace.com**.

Similar to meditation, *mindfulness* is something we have been hearing a lot about lately, not only in education circles but in the corporate world as well. Even this book uses the term *mindful moment* at the beginning of each chapter. So, what's the difference between meditation and mindfulness?

Opinions vary, but according to Andy Puddicombe, an ex-monk turned start-up entrepreneur who is behind the successful Headspace meditation app, the difference may be subtle yet important. Puddicombe sees the daily implementation of meditation as a means of attaining mindfulness—mindfulness meaning being present in the moment with an awareness as to what you're thinking, feeling, and experiencing in that moment (2011). According to other leading experts, mindfulness is a form of meditation. In any case, the terms are often used interchangeably, referring to the same practice—taking a moment to calm your mind and center your thoughts. Mindfulness tends to be the preferred secular term used in education settings. No matter the vernacular, we as adults need to be tuned in to our own emotions and behaviors that we bring into our learning environments as we begin to implement these practices for students. Let's explore some mindfulness strategies to consider incorporating into your professional practice.

My school has implemented a whole-school mindful moment practice. We ask all students, teachers, and guests to stop what they are doing and participate. Our librarian rings a chime at 9:15 every day and leads the school over the intercom in a mindful practice. Sometimes we are doing butterfly breathing, and other times we are just focusing on the in-and-out of our breath. Once we set the standard that this is something we do every day, it was normalized, and the kids love starting the day with this practice. I tell them, "give yourself the gift of relaxing and focus on yourself."

Environment over Method

According to Karen Pittman, co-founder of the Forum for Youth Investment and a leader in the SEL movement, an evolving area of research centered on the science of learning tells us that "in order for children and youth to learn specific content (academic or otherwise), we must first ensure that we have created learning environments in which they feel socially accepted, emotionally safe, and generally supported" (Pittman n.d.). Pittman places an emphasis on environment over method, meaning that rather than getting caught up in best practices and most effective strategies for teaching SEL, we should first focus on the environment we create as educators as the most important factor in fostering SEL skills in our students. Furthermore, Pittman asserts that learning, in and of itself, is a social and emotional activity. With this in mind, how do we begin to create an environment conducive to SEL skill-building?

Practicing Mindfulness

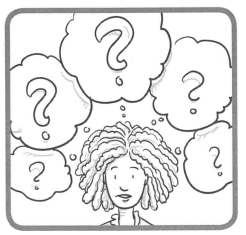
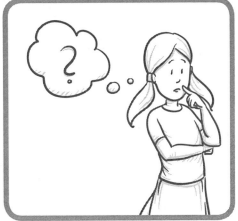

Begin by being mindful of exactly which emotions *you* are bringing into the classroom or learning environment each day when working with students. This can be achieved by a simple mental check-in or *mindful moment* with yourself. It's like taking your emotional temperature.

Implementing a *mindful moment* in your daily practice can then be expanded to include your students as well. At the start of each class or program, ask students to check in with themselves and take notice of what emotions they may be experiencing at that moment. Have students think about how these emotions might be impacting their behavior (positively or negatively).

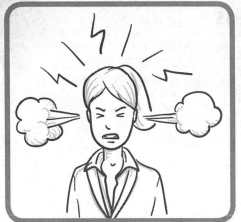 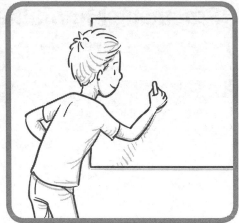

It is important to note that students should not be judging or punishing themselves when making connections between their emotions and behaviors. The focus of this practice should purely be on mindfulness. Exercise caution when having students share out their responses to ensure the necessary safe and supportive environment has been established.

You may have heard the phrase *name it to tame it*, which means being able to identify the emotion being experienced (name it) in order to manage the resulting behavior or reaction to it (tame it). This concept alone encapsulates virtually all five of CASEL's core competencies: self-awareness, self-management, social awareness, relationship skills, and responsible decision-making.

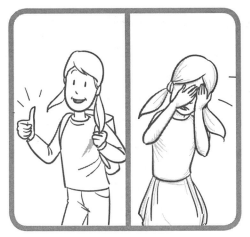

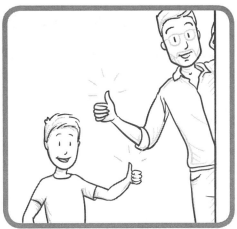

A similar check-in activity, Sunshine and Shadows, asks students to identify something they feel happy about and something they feel sad, anxious, or fearful about. The key to this type of exercise is helping students make the connection between the event, the emotion, and the resulting reaction or behavior exhibited. A step beyond this self-awareness is to then help guide students' thinking toward safe and healthy ways to manage their emotions and engage in responsible decision-making.

There are many different forms this practice can take and various methods and tools to utilize. Finding the right one for your individual practice and individual students may be a matter of trial and error. Remember, learning from failure is a good thing (provided you have cultivated the necessary foundation of trust among you and your students and among student peers in your learning environment).

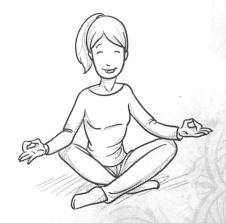

Teachers as Emotional Detectives

An alternative to a group check-in process (such as that used in Sunshine and Shadows) is to implement a confidential, student-to-teacher only check-in process. HelloYello, a web-based check-in system, was the brainchild of brothers and fellow special education teachers Brandon and Ryan Sportel (**www.helloyello.net**). In a 2015 article written by Brandon, he explains the genesis of HelloYello. While counseling a student on behavioral issues, he found himself asking the question all educators ask: "Why would you do something like that?" Then, he had an epiphany:

> "I had this realization that I was expecting the student [a fourth grader] to somehow psychoanalyze himself and come up with a grand justification for his behavior and actions. Asking the, 'why did you do it,' question did not help me to solve the issue—and I realized it never would. It was simply a fallback question for adults when they were not sure what to do" (Sportel 2015).

That light bulb moment inspired the Sportel brothers' creation of HelloYello. What they realized was that students needed a means of confidentially checking in with their teacher regarding their state-of-mind at any given moment, as well as an opportunity for self-reflection. They discovered that students were much more willing to be open and honest about their feelings when reporting through the app than in a face-to-face encounter.

Sportel goes on to explain, "Students with difficult behavior are not the only ones who struggle emotionally. Students often internalize feelings and lack the ability to express their needs appropriately, which makes it nearly impossible for teachers to recognize what is motivating their actions" (Sportel 2015). In terms of behavior issues, follow-up conversations between the teacher and student help the student connect the dots between their emotions and their behaviors and reflect on appropriate replacement behaviors to be applied in the future. In some cases, a student check-in might require a referral to a school counselor or administrator, as appropriate. By getting at the root emotion a child is experiencing, we are able to more effectively counsel them and provide them with acceptable replacement behaviors. Check-ins are not meant only for negative emotions; students are encouraged to report positive feelings as well, much like in Sunshine and Shadows. A sample student check-in (figure 3.3) and the HelloYello Reflection Form (figure 3.4) are shown below.

Figure 3.3 HelloYello Sample Check-In

I feel upset and sad because I think that it is not fair that only your groups can get homework passes but my group or toni's group don't get any and we behave (96% most of the time)

I think that you should ask zaiden's mom or sammie's mom how we did. If we can get home works passes I would appreciat it! thanks!

Figure 3.4 HelloYello Reflection Form

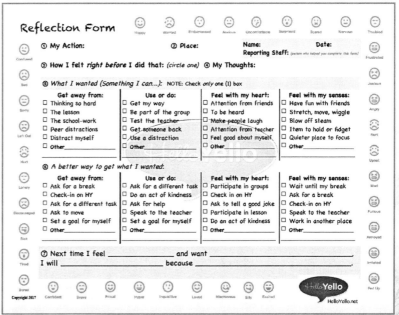

Through the HelloYello system, students report to their teacher on their emotional state-of-mind. A student check-in may be as simple as *I feel happy today because my soccer team won* or as serious as *I feel tired today because my parents were fighting last night and I couldn't sleep.* Then, at some point during the school day, the teacher will acknowledge each student's check-in with a brief face-to-face encounter (e.g., *Congratulations on your soccer win!* or *I'm sorry to hear you had a rough night last night. Would you like to talk about that?*) According to the data, this simple process goes a long way in building trusting and caring relationships between students and teachers, resulting in improved classroom climate as students become more apt to confide issues of bullying and other stressors that may be impeding their academic success. HelloYello is also able to capture classroom and school climate data (figure 3.5).

Figure 3.5 Sample School Climate Data from HelloYello

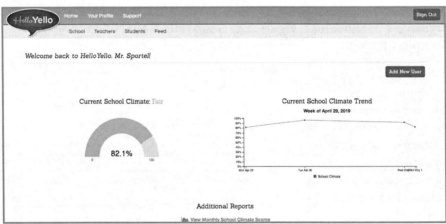

Managing Student Stress

SEL Spotlight: Trisha DiFazio
Adjunct Professor,
University of Southern California

I travel around the country talking to students to try and get a better idea of how to improve their social-emotional experience in schools. I always ask students, "What are three things that cause you stress in the classroom?" The number one named stressor of students? Cold calling—being called on when you do not have the answer is one of the most stressful experiences for students in grades K–8, so much so that students reported experiencing physical symptoms of stress by the mere sight or sound of the ubiquitous popsicle sticks. In the words of one fourth grader, "I didn't know the answer before the teacher called on me, and I'm not going to know the answer after." Oftentimes, calling on a student at random is used to draw attention to the fact that they are not paying attention. This practice is punitive and shame-based. Cold calling is especially harmful for English language learners as it does not allow for the wait time necessary to translate from their first language into their second. Cold calling at its core is meant to provide accountability and promote participation. However, students report that they feel embarrassed almost immediately. After many conversations, I discovered that students prefer "warm calling," meaning that they are allowed to do a think-pair-share and/or write-pair-share so they are equipped with an answer before being called at random. This lowers their affective filter and creates a sense of confidence. If you're ever curious about how your lessons are going or how to improve classroom climate, I encourage you to simply ask your bosses: the 30 faces staring at you.

Just like their teachers, students also experience stress. Research shows that moderate levels of stress are actually beneficial in developing resiliency in both children and adults. However, chronic or toxic stress, such as the type experienced by children of poverty, is shown to have a debilitating and enduring negative impact on student outcomes (Jensen 2009). Developing healthy coping mechanisms to manage stress is paramount to learning and achieving success. Resiliency research identifies the toxic stress that many at-risk and students of poverty experience as significantly contributing to their academic struggle (Walsh 2015). The term *at-risk* has been used to define students "who are likely to fail in school or in life because of their life's social circumstances" (Leroy and Symes 2001). This can be attributed to multiple factors, yet poverty is primary among them.

Students on the opposite end of the socioeconomic spectrum can also experience high levels of stress. "Children of affluence are generally presumed to be at low risk. However, recent studies have suggested problems in several domains—notably, substance use, anxiety, and depression—and two sets of potential causes: pressures to achieve and isolation from parents" (Luthar 2003). This reinforces the fact that *all* students need SEL. Educators must strive to create the environment necessary to support all students' social and emotional development.

One of the best visual depictions of how stress affects students' brains, emotions, and behaviors, and how practices such as deep breathing techniques and mindfulness can help, can be found in a video called *Just Breathe,* accessible from the Mindful Schools website (**www.mindfulschools.org/inspiration/just-breathe-julie-bayer-salzman/**).

The results speak for themselves. Here are a few quotes from both students and adults that have benefitted from mindfulness programs in their schools:

> "Students are coming to school with a variety of issues . . . poverty, dysfunctional home environments, homelessness. Some of our students don't have the same place to sleep every night. They couch surf or they move around a lot. They don't have that stability. We have quite a few students who are very depressed, and then we have a lot of students who are very angry . . . and then we have students who are sad, very sad. Before a student can actually learn in the classroom, we have to take care of the needs of the *person* first . . . if that's food, if that's a hug."
>
> —Morgan, Teacher

> "It really comes down to self-knowing, self-awareness. My goal is to give them experiences of learning about themselves . . . and coping mechanisms to develop resiliency. I would say at-risk students display the most grit [resiliency]—they have looked into the mouth of the dragon. But they often have the least amount of coping skills. For example, active listening is an SEL skill. And often, because they haven't been listened to, and they don't trust others will listen to them, it's just not a skill in practice for them."
>
> —Anna, Therapist

> "We have teen parents here. Sometimes they don't know how to deal with the stress. They can't relax at home because they have their kid to worry about."
>
> —Bill, Student, 18

"I have been practicing mindfulness with my students for three years now. Mindfulness is a mental state achieved by focusing one's own awareness on the present moment while calmly acknowledging and accepting one's feelings, thoughts, and bodily sensations. I needed a visual way for my students to understand what mindfulness was and the purpose it had. It all began with an activity from Mindfulness in After-school: A 16-Session Curriculum that involved a plastic water bottle filled with water and glitter. I showed them the still water bottle with the glitter resting at the bottom of it. I asked them if they were able to see through the water bottle, and of course, their response was 'yes' since the water was clear and calm. After I shook the entire water bottle, I then asked them again, 'Can you see through the water bottle now?' They all responded 'no' with such wonder in their eyes. I then explained to them how that water bottle was our brain and the glitter represented our thoughts. When I introduced mindfulness to them, I explained how it was a powerful tool to help us calm that glitter down in our brains so that we would be able to clear our minds in order to make wise decisions. They then understood how it all worked, and they were all motivated to calm their glitter."

—Erika Chavez, Program Leader

"Because after, you feel all peaceful and relaxed."

—Jared-James, Student, 19, on why he arrives at school an hour early to participate in a meditation group

Promising Practices for SEL Skill Development

Among the most important of my findings in my work with SEL, with which all experts I've spoken with have agreed, is that in order for students to master SEL skills, adults must walk them through the process of what they are learning while they are experiencing it. In other words, when students are expressing frustration, anxiety, or defeat, that is when the adult must step in and guide them through the process of what they are feeling, how that feeling manifests in their behaviors, and how to persevere through the challenge. This is how students learn to connect the dots between their emotions and their behaviors in a way that is relatable to the specific SEL skills they are working to develop. Moreover, adults can help kids see how these skills can be transferred to other settings and situations, making them relevant to their lives and future goals.

Although it is recommended that schools and programs adopt an evidenced-based SEL curriculum and framework, there is no one-size-fits all approach to SEL. Research informs us that everyone learns differently. SEL is no exception to that rule. SEL skills can be fostered through myriad activities, regardless of whether activities are specifically labeled as SEL. As Morgan, a teacher, commented, "It's not important why they are there but what is happening while they are there. The level of critical thinking . . . it grows into a really cool learning environment for those kids." Observations like these are substantiated by Duckworth's findings on the many ways in which students gain SEL skills through a variety of activities and experiences (2016).

Project-Based Learning

A key finding in my SEL programming experience, particularly for at-risk youth, is the discovery of the importance of group learning projects. As Anna, a therapist and SEL specialist, shared with me, "At-risk students, in particular, really prefer group projects, community projects, where there isn't too much pressure, but they can have ownership in the greater community. They much more easily give up on the individual projects. That's one of the strengths of having a social emotional component: to see this not as a negative but as a sign of their struggles." In other words, for vulnerable student populations in particular, cultivating SEL skills through collaborative projects and activities is an effective and supportive approach to learning.

Furthermore, this collaborative approach to learning is universally applicable to all students, as supported by the framework for twenty-first-century skills and the four Cs: critical thinking, communication, collaboration, and creativity. Additional support for this strategy can be found in *Preparing Youth to Thrive: Promising Practices for Social & Emotional Learning* (Smith et al. 2016). Most importantly, this community project approach to learning also promotes a sense of school connectedness, belonging, and engagement . . . or, as one principal simply termed it, "school spirit," further motivating students to attend and participate in school.

SEL Spotlight: Kris Hinrichsen
Teacher, Chinook Open Optional Program

My school has many opportunities for students in different grades to interact. We have a community garden that my class gets to plant and harvest each year. The upper grades get to water, chop, and cook the vegetables, and we have a yearly harvest soup in multi-age groups. The traditions my class gets to partake in help strengthen their connections to school and other students outside of our class.

Family Engagement and Cultural Inclusivity

In his book, *Culturally and Linguistically Responsive Teaching and Learning, Second Edition* (2018), Dr. Sharroky Hollie talks about the historical roots of the deculturalization of students in the American school system as contributing to systemic racism. *Deculturalization* is the practice of forced assimilation of students from all backgrounds in order to fit neatly into a one-size-fits-all institutionalized system. Our education system was largely structured according to the tenets of white, Christian culture. This speaks to why students from the culture that founded the system would naturally have an advantage over those from other cultures. Having educators come to recognize this more fully in recent years has resulted in greater efforts toward cultural awareness, acceptance, and inclusivity. However, we still have a long way to go toward a more equitable system that embraces and values all cultures. This is part of the reason we have seen more efforts to engage parents and families in education, along with the obvious acknowledgement that all parents have a vested interest in the quality of education their children receive—as well as the social and emotional culture their children experience in the course of their K–12 education.

In the past, there have been common misconceptions that parents from certain populations were less interested or less engaged in their children's education. However, a perceived lack of engagement may actually be a reflection of the cultural lens through which those parents' behavior is being viewed. Being actively engaged in a child's education may manifest in different ways and may vary from culture to culture. Additionally, many parents may feel alienated, intimidated, or disconnected from the school or community due to cultural or language barriers. This may inhibit their levels of comfort in participating in school events and conversations relating to their children's in-school experiences or academic performances. Along with the positive impact on students, SEL practices and activities may have the potential for increasing family engagement. With the implementation of ESSA, efforts toward greater family engagement have increased along with SEL strategies involving parents and families for a more holistic approach to education.

Many immigrant parents and families feel that because they themselves are not educated, they have nothing to offer or contribute to their child's education. This is sometimes misinterpreted by educators as parents being disengaged from their child's education. On the contrary, most immigrant families are very concerned about their kids not only getting a quality education but also about their well-being. Parents tend to undervalue their contributions in the way of social and emotional support. For example, a mom might view herself as not being very involved in her child's education because she is unable to assist with homework—yet, when you speak with her, she reveals she routinely provides food and treats for school events. From a cultural standpoint, this *is* family engagement!

Cultivating SEL through Extracurricular and After-School Activities

Extracurricular activities, including after-school and expanded learning programs (ELPs), are fertile ground for cultivating SEL skills. Unlike the traditional school day, these programs have long made SEL a top priority and enjoy the freedom and flexibility to do so, making ELPs an ideal environment for fostering SEL skill-building. In fact, Duckworth devotes an entire chapter of her 2016 book *Grit: The Power of Passion and Perseverance* to the virtues of extracurricular activities, such as sports, dance, and music as prime vehicles for the delivery of SEL skills. "There are countless research studies showing that kids who are more involved in extracurriculars fare better on just about every conceivable metric—they earn better grades, have higher self-esteem, are less likely to get in trouble, and so forth" (Duckworth 2016, 225). SEL in after-school activities and programs will be explored further in the following chapter.

Expanding Horizons: Cultivating a Growth Mindset

Creating opportunities for new experiences stimulates a growth mindset. Many students from low socioeconomic backgrounds and other high-risk populations are often limited in their scope of experience with people and perspectives that differ from their own cultures and communities. Enrichment activities, such as school field trips, provide an opportunity to capitalize on the SEL benefits and nuances such exposure can bring.

Broadening horizons through exposure to new experiences comes in many forms and impacts students in myriad aspects of their lives. Phil, a principal at a continuation high school with a high at-risk population and an integrated SEL program in both the instructional day and after school, says that many of his students have an interest in becoming a probation officer, a therapist, or a counselor. Although these are all noble professions, Phil describes a lack of exposure to other professions as the reason for these choices. "These are the people who have impacted them along the way and have shaped their experience, so these are the occupations they know about." This was reinforced in my conversations with high school students, Ruby and Bill, both 18. Ruby shared with me that she wanted to be a mediator, like the one she interacted with during her parents' divorce and custody battle. And Bill told me that even though his friends don't like cops, he wanted to be a police officer because he had "seen a lot of bad stuff go down" and he wanted to stay on the right side of the law. While these are certainly valid career choices, it does speak to Phil's point about students aspiring to professions with which they are familiar. Another educator at the same school site echoed a similar sentiment: "Our students get outside their communities very little. We try to get students to leave their comfort zone, get out of their little box, and really experience something different." Whether they go on to college, students can benefit from experiences that expand their horizons and develop their SEL skill sets. Even incorporating guest speakers from diverse backgrounds, personally and professionally, can make a huge impact on a student's perspective and mind-set.

In other words, a focus on SEL through enrichment opportunities has the potential to fill the void marginalized students might be experiencing. Participating in learning activities that take place beyond the classroom walls broadens their scope of what's possible for their futures, keeping them engaged and motivated to learn and achieve.

"I think of the kids in our programs, [low socioeconomic, at-risk students] who have not had the chance to be exposed to 'what's possible.' . . . We target those kids who really have not had the opportunities that a lot of other kids have had growing up."

— Michael Funk, Director of the Expanded Learning Division at the California Department of Education

SEL Spotlight: Ernesto Durán
Regional Lead, CDE
Expanded Learning Division

Transitioning to an affluent suburb in the U.S. from Mexico City was culture shock, to say the least. I entered school in California at age 13, having only completed through third grade in Mexico. However, I quickly caught up to my peers, primarily due to three factors: high academic expectations; a support system; and having my social and emotional needs met. Many classrooms are not student-centered and offer students very few opportunities to interact and build their language skills. As a newcomer, I learned most of my English not in the classroom, but on the playground.

Summary

Creating a healthy, happy environment begins with the adults working in that environment. School settings and the education process itself are often riddled with stress. Implementing ways to mitigate stress in both adults and students is paramount to creating effective learning environments. As educators, the best starting point for creating this environment is with our own SEL practice and in being *mindful* of the emotions and behaviors we bring into our educational settings each day. Additionally, creating effective SEL learning environments extends beyond the classroom walls, from establishing safe home environments for students to expanding students' horizons through field trips and after-school programs.

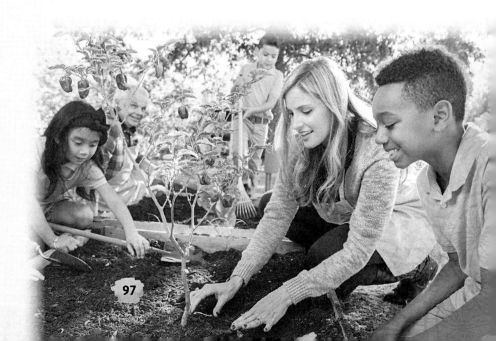

Points to **Ponder**

1. After reading this chapter, how have your responses to the pre-reading questions changed? Do you feel you have a better grasp on what it means to create a SEL environment? What questions remain?

2. What is meant by the phrase *environment over method*?

3. What do you envision as the ideal environment for SEL to thrive?

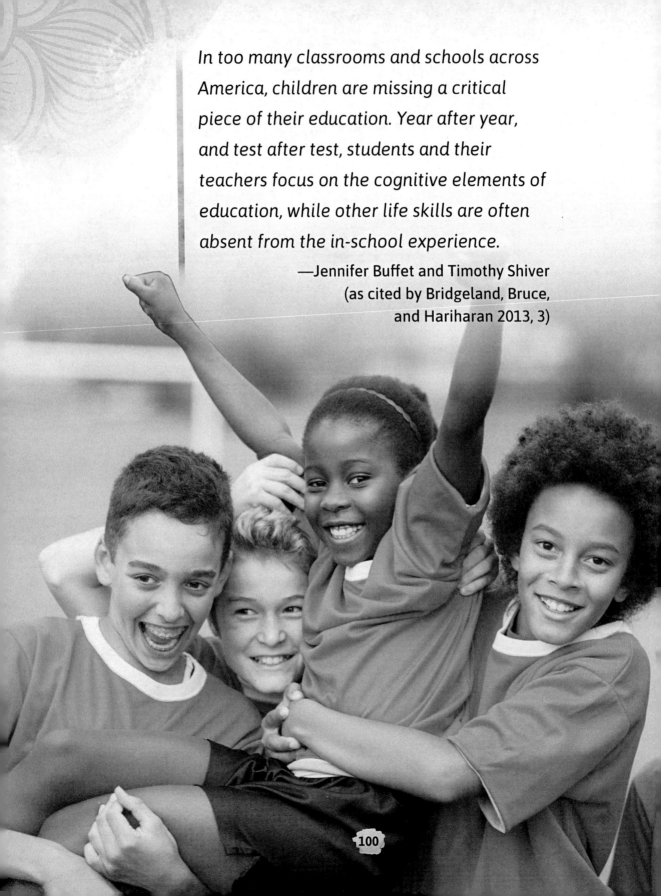

In too many classrooms and schools across America, children are missing a critical piece of their education. Year after year, and test after test, students and their teachers focus on the cognitive elements of education, while other life skills are often absent from the in-school experience.

—Jennifer Buffet and Timothy Shiver
(as cited by Bridgeland, Bruce, and Hariharan 2013, 3)

Chapter Four

Learning
Doesn't Stop at the Bell:
SEL After School

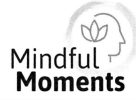

Mindful
Moments

* What, if any, extracurricular or after-school activities are available to your students?

* Is SEL addressed (either directly or indirectly) during these activities?

* How can an extracurricular or after-school activity support in-class SEL skill development?

As a child, did you participate in sports or dance? Did you take art classes? Did you take piano lessons or play another instrument? Did you sing in the church choir or march in the school band? Were you a member of the yearbook committee, debate team, or student leadership? Or were you involved in academic pursuits, such as the science club or mock trial? Were you involved in community service projects?

Before you start to feel like an underachiever, here's my confession: I did none of these extracurricular activities. I wish I had. Had I felt more connected to school, perhaps I would have been motivated to engage in such activities. But thinking back to Maslow's Hierarchy of Needs, kids need to have their basic needs met before they can aspire to higher-level goals. I just wasn't there yet. I was in survival mode. By the time I got to high school, I needed to get a job. I worked after school and on weekends. The workplace became my escape and where I obtained most of my SEL skills.

In an ideal world, children should have the opportunity to grapple with real-world challenges *and* the opportunity to discover their passions through engaging in activities that are meaningful to them. Some kids from hardscrabble backgrounds find their escape in school, which is a healthy and productive coping mechanism. But others are like me—they disengage, and in some cases, they drop out altogether. Educators can help their students discover their passions—a surefire way to keep them motivated and engaged in school.

For students without the family resources to participate in many of the enrichment activities enjoyed by their wealthier peers, sponsored after-school programs become their extracurriculars. The programs provide them with opportunities to expand their horizons and to develop their SEL skill set, and they may provide additional academic support as well.

According to a 2014 report from the Afterschool Alliance entitled "America After 3PM," 10.2 million children, or 18 percent of the national K–12 population, participate in publicly funded after-school and expanded learning programs. Students who attend regularly stand to gain upward of 90 additional school days per year. Imagine the potential impact of that additional time and support, particularly for marginalized students who are typically the participants of such programs. Perhaps even more important is the access to the enrichment activities these programs provide, designed to expand horizons and foster SEL skill development—important factors in addressing the opportunity/achievement gap. The additional time afforded to students participating in these programs is one thing, but it is what we do with that time that matters.

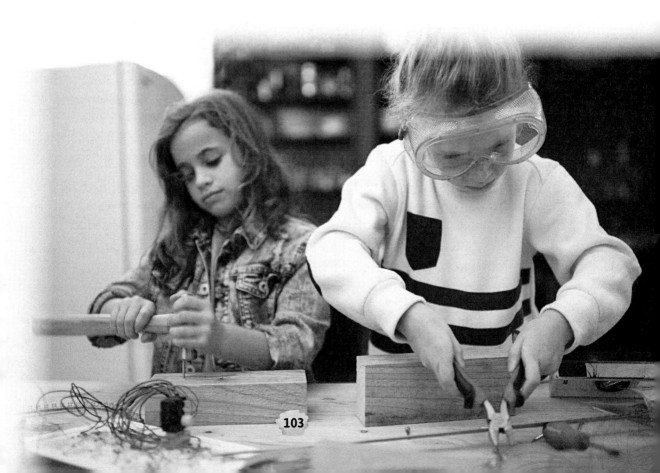

SEL in Action: What Does It Look Like?

Navigating SEL from the Inside Out documents a look inside 25 leading SEL programs. An excerpt from the report, published by the Harvard Graduate School of Education, explains the purpose and need for this resource: "In our work as researchers and educators, our team frequently receives questions about the content, implementation, and effectiveness of SEL programs and interventions. While good resources exist to identify evidence-based programs (see CASEL's guides, 2003, 2013, 2015), there are currently no available resources to help stakeholders look inside these programs to see how they differ from one another and what makes each program unique" (Jones et al. 2017, 4).

While it is recommended you implement evidenced-based curricula in your practice, highlighted in this chapter are ways in which you can begin to explore and capitalize on the SEL benefits inherently embedded in common activities. In our own experience with implementing SEL programming, primarily in after-school programs, we have discovered that there is no one-size-fits-all approach to SEL. Every program, school community, and student population is unique and deserves to be treated as such. However, some opportunities to tap into SEL skills are more obvious than others. Years ago, our expanded learning programs began with yoga, meditation, and mindfulness. Although these were incredibly popular, successful, and impactful experiences for students, we soon realized this is not the only road to SEL. We discovered SEL was hiding all around us. We began to investigate the potential of other activities and programming to see if in fact educators and students might be "doing SEL" without even realizing it. Sure enough, many were.

This was an important discovery for us and may be for you as well. You may find you already have programs in place that you have not yet recognized as having the potential to provide SEL skill development, or you may just not be intentionally utilizing that potential. For example, in our practice, we stumbled upon several different organizations that thought they were offering one thing but were offering much more than they realized. The following sections provide examples of the many forms SEL might take.

Giving Kids WINGS

WINGS for Kids is one of only three after-school programs listed in the previously mentioned report on the top 25 SEL programs (2017). WINGS has been on the SEL scene since 1996, providing comprehensive SEL programming for students in grades K–5 in *out-of-school time* settings. The program focuses on building healthy relationships between children and adults and promoting positive behaviors and responsible decision-making. The curriculum consists of weekly lesson plans that are SEL skill-set specific and that span the course of the school year. Activities include community-building and service-learning projects as well as role-playing and discussion to help students connect the dots between their emotions and behaviors. Lessons are structured in scope and sequence and allow for flexibility of local adaptation.

Based in North Carolina with program sites around the country, WINGS operates its programs as a comprehensive pilot site model, meaning it's much more than just curriculum: it's the whole package. I had the pleasure of observing several WINGS lessons and strategies in action at their West Coast pilot schools. I observed the activity described below, which was designed to connect students with specific emotions and help them recognize such emotions in themselves and in others. This is just one example of an activity that helps create an effective SEL environment.

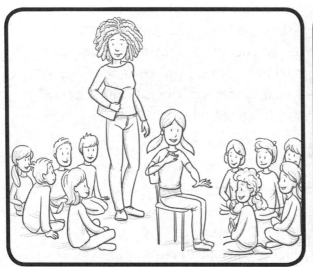

The teacher sits in the center of the room while students sit in a circle on the floor surrounding her or him. One student volunteer sits in a chair next to the teacher facing toward the class.

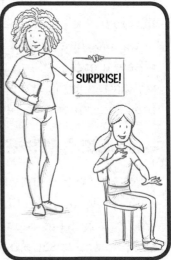

The teacher holds up a sign (behind the line of vision of the volunteer) on which an emotion was written, for example, *surprise*.

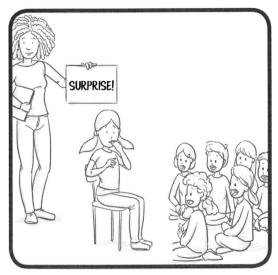

The class silently reads the emotion being shown and then demonstrates the emotion with body language and facial expressions.

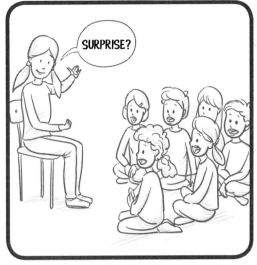

Based on how the class interprets the emotion, the student volunteer guesses which emotion their peers are trying to express.

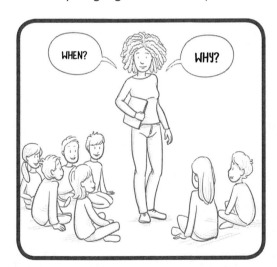

The teacher may also share examples or engage in a conversation about when and why each emotion might be expressed, to deepen students' learning around each concept.

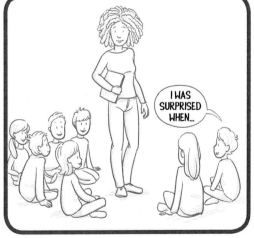

As a closing activity, the teacher goes around the circle using a talking stick to have each student make a statement about one of the emotions covered in the day's lesson. These simple statements can be used by the teacher in encouraging students to think about the emotion on a deeper level.

Students were enthusiastically engaged and eager to participate in both roles, as the expresser and as the guesser. Through this activity, students can learn to recognize emotions through self-expression and pro-socialization. Students now have an opportunity to expand on their vocabulary, deepen the connection to their emotions, and better understand how those emotions affect their behaviors.

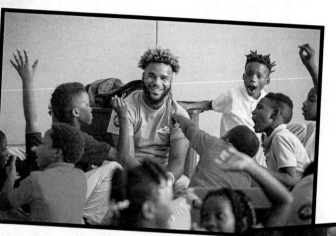

This teacher had cultivated an environment in which all students felt safe and comfortable in expressing their feelings and emotions with their peers—a prerequisite for implementing these types of activities.

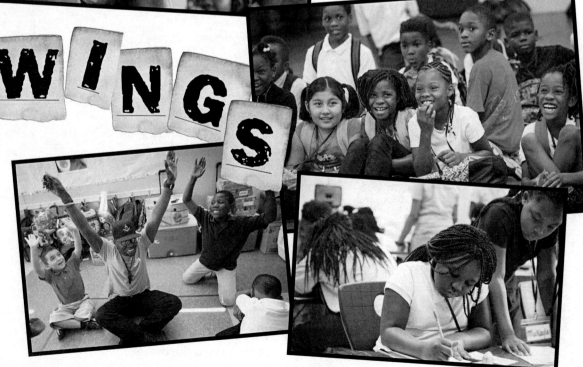

Beyond Yoga and Mindfulness

My philosophy around SEL programming is grounded in the theory that, just as with academics, every student learns through a different modality, and each has a different interest and way in which they find meaning and relevance in their learning. With this in mind, we began implementing and observing learning environments that embraced this concept and integrated SEL strategies in a number of innovative ways.

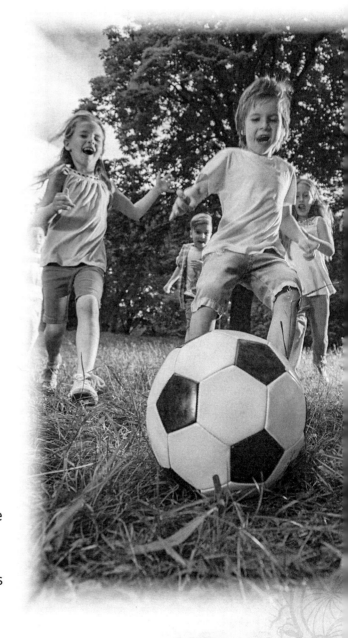

Through case study observations and anecdotal data, our findings align with existing research that supports activities such as sports, dance, and the arts as prime curricula to infuse essential SEL skill-building lessons. In most cases, students are naturally being exposed to SEL skills as a side effect of participating in these types of activities. Imagine the potential impact on student outcomes with the implementation of *intentionality* in practice. Starting with activities where we already know SEL is lurking, ready and waiting to be seized upon, will get us closer to our instructional goals as quickly as possible.

Sports—The SEL No-Brainer

Any athlete, coach, or virtually anyone who has participated in sports can identify the SEL skills developed as a result of that experience: teamwork, sportsmanship, positive attitude, determination, resiliency, and grit are among them. This is why I call sports the "no-brainer" of SEL. However, many sports programs, or the schools and youth organizations that use them, fail to capitalize on the SEL potential with intentionality.

We implemented a soccer program, the creators of which recognized they were teaching much more than soccer (and we chose that program over others for that reason). Once a week, the soccer coach would come prepared to infuse the fun on the field with meaningful and impactful lessons on vital SEL skills. I recall observing a lesson on respect, in which the coach used time-outs and water breaks to infuse the concept of respect and how it applies to teammates on the field as well as to teachers and parents. These fourth and fifth graders enthusiastically engaged in conversations about how they show respect for others. When the coach asked for an example of how to show respect for parents or caregivers while at home, one student offered, "You should eat what they make you for dinner even if you don't like it." Encouraging students to transfer their learning around SEL skills to other circumstances is an important aspect of SEL instruction.

As impressive as this was to watch in action, how do we know it's really making a lasting impact on students and not just for the hour or two each week when the coach is present? One way to ensure a lasting impact is to reinforce these lessons throughout the week and beyond. For example, during an activity unrelated to soccer, a program facilitator might ask students to recall and reflect on the lesson the coach taught the previous week and how it applies to a different activity or situation. When staff members reinforce the lesson, students are given additional opportunities to reflect on the lesson and to practice applying the skills learned in different settings and circumstances. This ensures the skills learned are transferrable, which is an important aspect in SEL skill development. The particular soccer program we implemented, Mighty Kicks, is only available locally in Southern California. However, other programs, such as the U.S. Soccer Foundation, are available nationwide. For more information, visit their website at **www.ussoccerfoundation.org**.

During the traditional school day, similar opportunities for SEL skill development can be found during P.E. for secondary education or during recess for elementary settings.

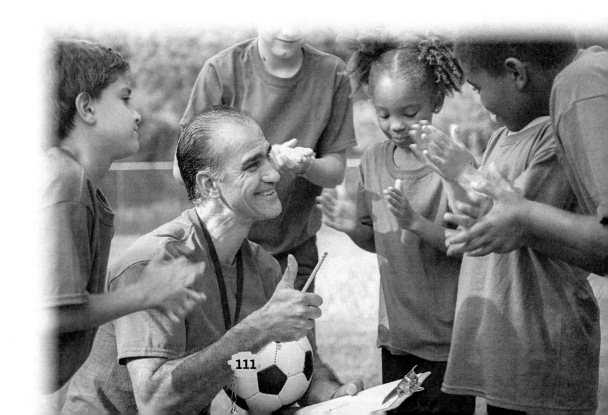

SEL Spotlight: Kris Hinrichsen
Teacher, Chinook Open Optional Program

One of the biggest opportunities to practice SEL is at recess, when there are 125 kids and only four adults. I make a regular practice of doing a recess debrief when the class gets back. Early in the year, there are lots of things to talk about: how the tools we have learned for managing emotions and interactions are, or are not, working. We get to redo and role-play how we would do things differently if they came up again. The key is that the kids are learning the skills, and I am teaching them how to approach solving problems. When students can self-identify as problem solvers, they will work much harder at solving problems. If adults in their lives always swoop in to solve their problems, students come to believe they are not capable of solving their own problems. This results in more tattling in the classroom and less development of SEL skills.

Another fantastic sports program for promoting SEL skills is the First Tee's DRIVE program. Educators may wonder whether golf would widely appeal to their students, but students who are unfamiliar with the sport have the added benefit of exposure to a new experience.

The acronym DRIVE stands for Develops Rewarding, Inspiring Values for Everyone. The DRIVE program aligns the First Tee's golf curriculum with SEL competencies, such as interpersonal skills, self-management, and resiliency. Operating under nine core values, the curriculum connects the positive attributes of golf with valued personal characteristics, such as honesty, respect, perseverance, and courtesy. See the First Tee's website for more information: **www.thefirsttee.org**.

Everybody Dance Now!

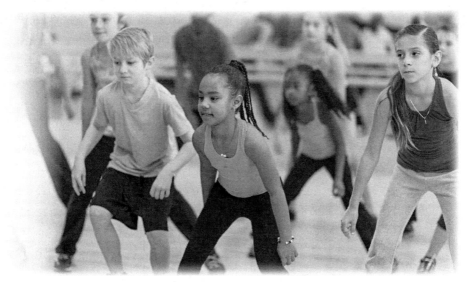

In the closing chapter of this book, you will read about a young
girl named Jackie who started a nonprofit organization at age 12.
Everybody Dance Now! (EDN) was established locally and has since
grown into a nationwide organization, bringing the joy of hip-hop
dance to students who might not otherwise have access to such
enrichment opportunities. Although the creators of EDN originally saw
the program as merely a dance program, I realized it was much more
than that. SEL was hiding everywhere in a curriculum that teaches
students not only to dance but to learn and appreciate the diversity
and beauty of other cultures. Lessons are infused with bits of history,
geography, the arts, vocabulary, and other academic content areas
in the context of learning the historical origins and cultural roots of
various dance forms.

I have witnessed firsthand how kids blossom and grow in confidence
and self-esteem while learning to create a safe and supportive
environment for their peers and themselves where they can feel free
to express themselves through movement. Watching shy, introverted

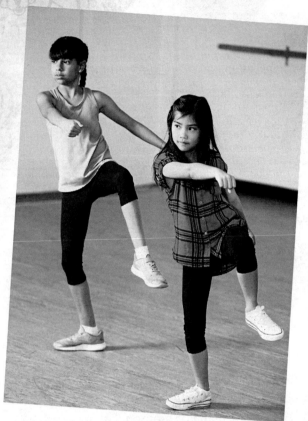

kids grow into self-confident and creative dancers (and students) is a testament to the impact of infusing SEL competencies into these types of programs. Of course, the right instructors, which EDN is careful to select, are paramount to the success of any program. Having adults who know and understand that they are teaching more than just dance, or soccer, or golf, or any academic subject for that matter, is key to cultivating SEL within any program. Visit EDN's website to learn more about bringing this valuable resource to your school or program: **www.everybodydancenow.org**.

All the same principles and SEL skills can be cultivated within any sports program implemented in your school or community program. The most important feature is adults who know to apply SEL with intentionality and who provide students with opportunities to practice and apply the transferrable skills developed on the soccer field, golf course, dance floor, etc. to other activities and experiences in their lives.

Our education system is very linear. However, life seldom is. Particularly for at-risk kids, following a traditional linear education path is difficult to do when your life is full of zigs and zags, detours, and crises. Most kids, whose lives aren't linear and are forced to fit into a uniform learning environment, have a hard time adapting and connecting to school. This is where after-school programs, which tend to be less restrictive and more fluid environments, can become the bridge that connects these students to their schools. I have spoken with countless students who tell me that the highlight of their day is their time spent in their after-school program. It is there that they forge meaningful relationships with their peers and with program staff members, who are closer to their age, grew up and live in the community, and who look like them.

It Takes a Village: Making an Impact through Service Learning

WE Schools is a global nonprofit organization offering free K–12 service learning curriculum that is accessible to all. WE Schools founder Craig Kielburger was also a mere 12-year-old when he began his nonprofit organization, then known as Free the Children. In his 2018 book, *WEconomy*, Kielburger explains the catalyst for his preteen charity venture. One morning, as he pulled the comics from the newspaper, he was struck by a photo of a young boy accompanied by the headline, "Battled child labor, boy, 12, murdered" (Kielburger, Branson, and Kielburger 2018, 32). He describes the impact he felt reading that the boy, Iqbal, was the same age as him. "Until that moment, my life had been pretty ordinary. . . . I didn't know it then, but Iqbal had just changed the course of my life. As I stared back at that photo of Iqbal, I knew I wanted to help other kids like him" (33). Young Kielburger's empathy for this boy, worlds apart from his own life experience, launched him into a lifelong endeavor to make the world a better place through service to others less fortunate than himself.

Kielburger set about enlisting the aid of his middle school peers in his crusade against child labor. What began as a school project has grown into a charitable empire championed by the likes of Richard Branson and Oprah Winfrey. Craig's organization went on to develop WE Villages, which supports sustainability in third-world communities, and WE Schools, which provides free curriculum that encourages students of all ages and backgrounds to get involved in service learning projects, both locally and globally, that inspire them in the way Iqbal inspired Craig.

The WE model is student-centered, with kids themselves selecting one local and one global community service project or cause that is important to them and their communities. Then, they raise awareness and advocacy through specific efforts determined by the students. In addition

"Service learning is an excellent instructional method for building character, developing effective social skills, understanding the perspectives of others, and developing students' self-confidence that they can make a difference in the world" (Elias and Arnold 2006, 50).

to helping others through such endeavors, students are exposed to myriad ways of discovering their interests and passions and finding meaning and purpose in engaging in the world around them.

The benefits gained through service learning encompass the full spectrum of emotions and the entire range of SEL core competencies, connecting students with compassion, empathy, humility, and gratitude as well as social-awareness, relationship skills, and responsible decision-making. Additionally, students engaged in service learning exhibit "improved acceptance of cultural diversity, service leadership, civic attitudes and volunteer behavior, and reduced engagement in risky behaviors"(Miyamoto 2015).

Service learning exposes students to the issues of the world, both locally and globally, and teaches them how they can become an instrument for positive social change. We have worked with the WE Schools service-learning curriculum in several after-school programs. Educator testimonials from one program are provided below and on the following page. It is important to note that the students from this program are not from affluent backgrounds. On the contrary, more than one-third of this student population lives below the poverty line. Yet they experienced ways they can contribute to making the world a better place for all.

> "We have been working with the WE Schools program for two years now, and every year it gets better and better. The students are responsible for planning the activities to earn our way to WE Day."
>
> After-School Program Site Leader

"For Christmas, we went to our local convalescent facility and sang to our elderly. We also brought them gifts that we made. When we came back, we shared our feelings on the experience. One student cried because an elderly person told her 'it was the first gift she had received in a long time.' This made the students realize that some of the elderly never have visitors."

After-School Program Activity Leader

"We created Easter baskets for the kids at the children's hospital. Our goal was to make 50 baskets, but we ended up with more than 100. The students were super excited they exceeded their goal!"

After-School Program Site Leader

"Participating in WE taught students that even the smallest contributions can make a big difference. Students collected change to buy goats for villages in Kenya. Their goal was to raise $50 for one goat, but after learning from the WE Schools videos about the huge impact only $50 and one goat can make, they were excited to exceed their goal. We ended up raising $150 and buying three goats!"

After-School Program Site Coordinator

"My students shared with me that WE Day inspired them to continue making a difference in our community and showed them that they are part of something bigger. They already have ideas for next year! They are proud to be part of the ME to WE movement, and to be recognized and appreciated for their efforts. Together, WE can make a difference."

After-School Program Site Leader

Students completing the required number of service hours, as verified by their teacher or program leader, are invited to attend a culminating celebratory event known as WE Day, a star-studded extravaganza held in multiple major cities across the nation and internationally. This is an event I have attended more than once alongside colleagues and students, and it is something you (and more importantly, your students) will never forget!

The Los Angeles WE Day has over 15,000 students show up each year to celebrate their successes with the likes of Selena Gomez, Jennifer Aniston, and Oprah Winfrey. In addition to celebrities, the day is filled with inspirational speakers and humanitarian heroes applauding the students' efforts to make the world a better place through community service, civic engagement, and social responsibility—shifting from a ME to WE mindset, as the name implies. Featured speakers from the 2018 L.A. event included the student activists from Parkland, Florida. These student activists are an inspirational testament to the power of young people engaging in civil discourse, actively participating in democratic society, and applying what they have learned in school to real-world issues. WE Day events are also held in New York,

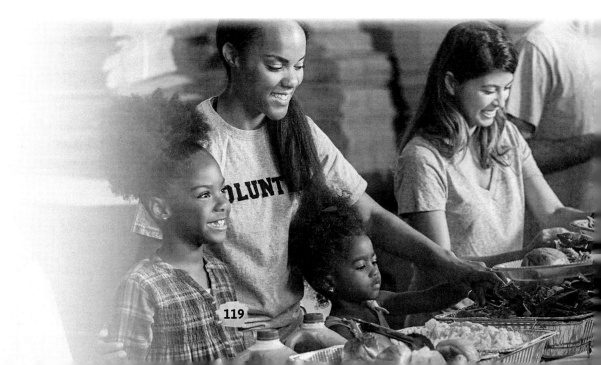

Chicago, Houston, and other major cities across the country as well as internationally, such as London and Toronto. Although the WE Day celebratory event is intended for older youth (middle and high school), service learning curriculum is adaptable for all ages and grade-spans. In fact, it is never too early to introduce the concept of service learning to students. For real-life examples of service learning projects for students as young as kindergarten, I highly recommend reading the "Vignettes of Service Learning and SEL in Action" featured in *The Educator's Guide to Emotional Intelligence and Academic Achievement* (Elias and Arnold 2006).

Because of the impact we've seen on our participating students, we have made extra efforts to provide resources and transportation to enable students from far-reaching rural areas to be able to attend the event. However, the experience of service learning alone, regardless of whether students attend the WE Day event, has been profound. Service learning projects can easily be implemented locally, and the SEL benefits naturally embedded can have a lifelong impact on students entering adult society with a sense of compassion and purpose. You can visit their website at **www.we.org**.

STEAM-SEL Connections

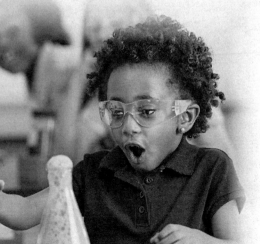

There is significant momentum around STEAM curricula, and this content is served well by project-based learning models. As Dr. Rebeca Andrade of Glendale Unified School District discovered, Expanded Learning Programs are also an "ideal ecosystem" for STEAM. Glendale USD has partnered with Piper (**www.playpiper. com**), an organization whose mission is to inspire the next generation of inventors, to help bring a makerspace feeling to their after-school program. Students are guided through design thinking and work together to actually build and code fully functioning computers. They ultimately build digital fluency while intentionally growing SEL skills, such as problem-solving, perseverance, and collaboration.

SEL through Family Engagement

SEL skill development through family engagement activities is an underdeveloped opportunity for infusing SEL with intentionality. This is also an area that is best developed locally, as every school community is different in terms of culture and demographics.

Principles & Parables: Correspondence Between Grandfather and Grandson (2016), a beautiful and insightful collection of letters on life lessons from lifelong educator Stan Seidman, was the inspiration for launching Lessons Involving Family Engagement (or LIFE Lessons). During the span of his 60-year career (yes, you read that correctly—60 years in education!), Principal Seidman worked with students and school environments on both ends of the socioeconomic spectrum. Seidman shares his vast experience, knowledge, and life lessons learned in the form of touching letters written to his grandson, Jaden. Although not intentional on the part of the author, I was struck by the SEL alignment evident in the messages contained in the letters. I found myself thinking, *Wouldn't it be great if every child had someone in their life to impart such wisdom?* To make it culturally relevant to our predominately Latino student population, I worked with Seidman to adapt and translate the book. LIFE Lessons (currently in development) includes projects such as interviewing family members about how they cope with stress or make tough decisions and about how they deal with sorrow and defeat. The interviews are discussed with peers and teachers to help connect the dots on the SEL skills that students' family members shared.

Using the WRITE Side of Your Brain

Another great SEL resource to utilize is Write Brain Books (**www.writebrainbooks.com**). Write Brain delivers SEL through multiple avenues, including academic content, project-based learning, family engagement, and creative arts, just to name a few. The curriculum is research-based, and it is aligned to college- and career-ready standards. Write Brain Books are wordless children's books in which the students themselves write the text. They become the storytellers, and ultimately, the published authors of their own books. An excerpt from their website explains:

> According to the theory of left-brain or right-brain dominance, each side of the brain controls different types of thinking. A child's right brain is activated when engaged in creative writing! . . . Resilience, creativity, flexibility, intuition, and intentionality are all skills that will increase their effectiveness in their lives. Life's difficulties will be easier to navigate. If young people understand how to think and to integrate emotion with analysis for problem solving, they will have an emotional intelligence that will pay off throughout their lives.

Another wonderful thing about this program is that it is adaptable for any age or grade. Although the books are illustrated as children's

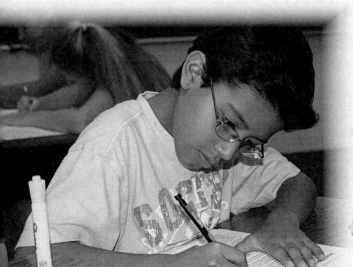

stories, they can be used with older students with the instruction that they are being asked to write a story for younger children. I also love the flexibility in that this can be done either as an individual activity or as a group project. My favorite part about the whole process is that in the end, each student completes the program with a published copy of their own book, listing them as the author! And to really put a finishing touch on the end product, a family engagement piece can be added by hosting a culminating activity in which the students participate in a book-signing event. Families attend to recognize their child's accomplishment of becoming a published author.

SEL through Acting and Improvisation

An area gaining traction and popularity as an effective vehicle for fostering SEL skill development is found in theater arts, more specifically through improvisation, or "improv" as it is commonly known. This is an area I have dabbled in with great success and plan to explore more extensively in the future. The rules of improv lend themselves to SEL because improv is all about listening skills—listening to what is said and then building on it. Practicing improv skills requires students to think on their feet, use their imagination, and be creative in a fun, fast-paced, and engaging way. Write Brain Books, the resource highlighted in the previous section, offers a free Improv curriculum.

As we know from movies and television, the use of comedy and drama can be an effective means of depicting the emotions and behaviors involved in real-life scenarios and relationships. Have you ever noticed how sometimes actors can be quite introverted and shy when not hiding behind a character, such as on a talk show or in an interview when they are not playing someone other than themselves? Taking on the role of a character enables them to more freely express emotions, such as anger, jealousy, or fear. Role-playing can allow students to put themselves in another's shoes, which is a great (and safe) way to express vulnerable emotions, such as empathy, sadness, or rejection.

One way to find instructors with the skill set needed to work with kids in acting and improv is through your local college or community theater group or even high-school drama clubs. We brought in a group of Theater Arts majors from a university to work with students from fourth through eighth grade in one of our after-school programs, and it was a huge hit! There's something about the energy of young people working with young people, particularly in this realm, that just really works. It's also an opportunity for children, sometimes living in isolated rural communities, to be exposed to subject matter they may not otherwise experience, and to have older students, particularly college students, as role models and mentors to inspire and excite them about the possibilities for their future. . . . Who knows, you may even discover the next Bryan Cranston!

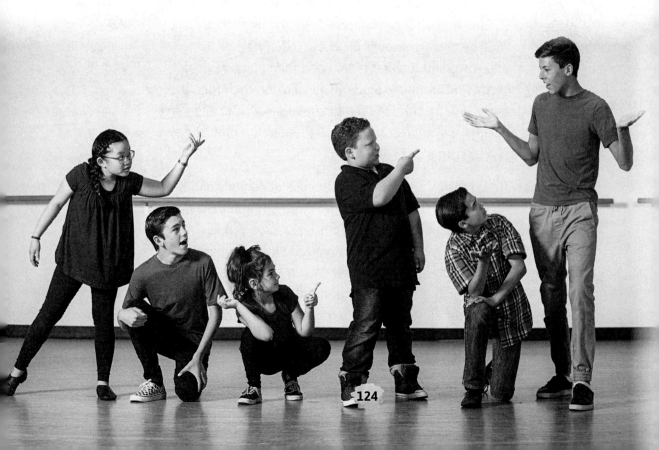

Summary

Although there is no one-size-fits-all approach to SEL, extracurricular activities and after-school programming are low-hanging fruit for SEL skill development, provided we are intentional in fostering and capitalizing on those opportunities. With some exceptions, such as WINGS for Kids and WE Schools, many of the programs and curricula highlighted in this chapter were discovered locally, and we worked collaboratively with those programs to cultivate and maximize the SEL potential. We do not purport to advocate for these homegrown SEL activities as being examples of evidence-based programs. That being said, based on our own firsthand experience, we can attest to the positive student impact we have witnessed as a result of their implementation. Most important is the acknowledgment that there are many different avenues for engaging kids in social and emotional skill-building . . . All roads lead to SEL!

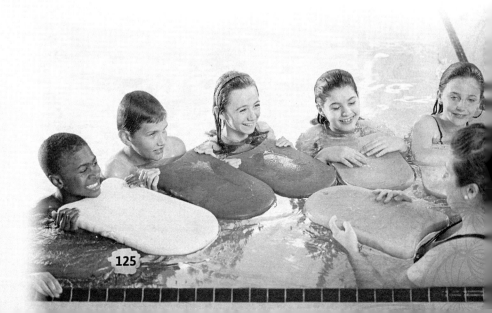

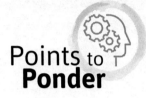

Points to
Ponder

1. Are there any extracurricular activities that your school, program, or community offers that could benefit from adding a SEL component?

_____

_____

_____

_____

_____

_____

_____

_____

_____

_____

_____

_____

_____

_____

_____

_____

_____

_____

2. What kinds of things does each program have in common?

_____

_____

_____

_____

_____

_____

_____

_____

3. How do you know if a program is impactful in terms of SEL?

_____

_____

_____

_____

_____

_____

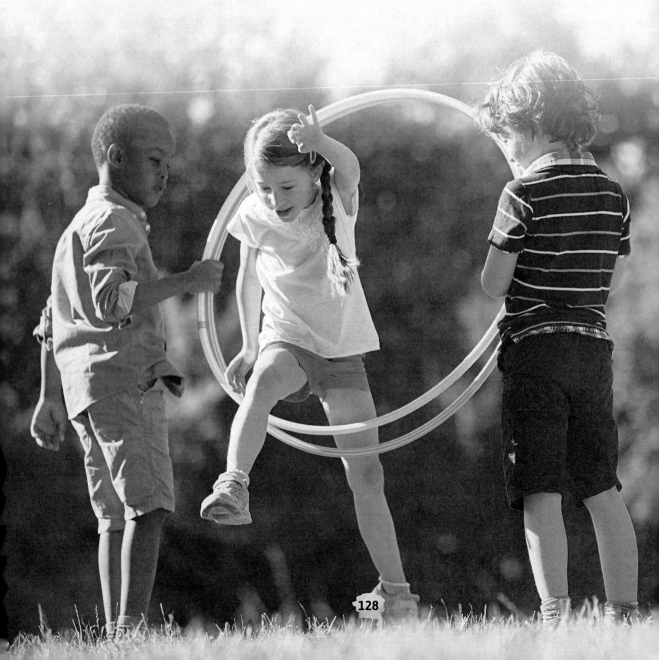

Education is what remains after one has forgotten what one has learned in school.

—Albert Einstein

Chapter Five

Redefining Student Success: SEL's Long-Term Impact

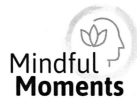

Mindful Moments

As you embark on the final chapter of this book, reflect on your answers to the following questions:

* How do you define student success?

* How do you envision the long-term impact of SEL in K–12 education?

* How might you begin to collect SEL data to help inform and refine your practice?

When educators relay student success stories, the story begins with a student overcoming challenges in their life, and it ends, more often than not, with the student graduating from a highly regarded university. And at the end of this book, you will find those types of student success stories. But in the course of my research on SEL, when I asked educators for their student success stories, what I got was something quite different. When I asked Dr. Jennifer Freed, a leading expert practitioner of SEL, for a student success story, here's what she shared with me:

"A boy who was in our [SEL] program in high school ran up to me on the street 10 or 12 years later. I almost didn't recognize him. He said, 'I'm so happy to see you. I'm a professional roofer, I have a wife and two babies. I'm so happy because every day I teach them what you taught me [SEL skills]. We talk to each other. I have a great life.'"

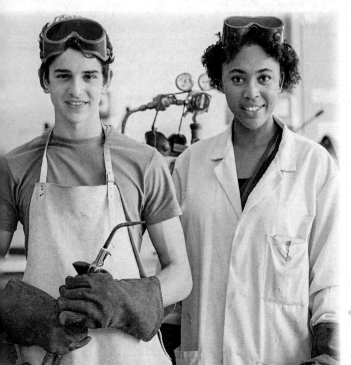

Similarly, Michael Funk, Director of the Expanded Learning Division of the CDE, shared with me his student success story. He said, "I think the most powerful student success story, for high school students, is when they find success in a career pathway because of their relationship with an educator." Referring to his own son's relationship with a science teacher, Funk said the following:

> "When he was going through one of his most difficult struggles, he reached out to that teacher, and the teacher wrote him a very powerful letter of recommendation and it really flipped the switch for him. He went from a kid who was afraid to interview for a job to one who's now thriving as a young manager of a business."

Funk went on to say that, as a parent, lots of things were helpful, but it took one of his son's high school educators to really "flip the switch" and facilitate that understanding. Funk's testimony speaks to key issues in education and also aligns with research that supports the positive impact of caring adult relationships on student outcomes.

What can be learned from these unique types of student success stories in support of the SEL movement going forward? Firstly, we must put an end to the belief that college is the one and only path to an individual's happiness and success in life. This sentiment was voiced by Dr. Freed:

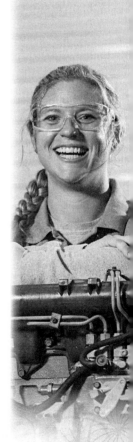

> "Why is it that we keep going cradle to college? We need people who are skilled at many, many different things. If I help someone gain the skills to become a good roofer [referring to her former student], a good mechanic, or a successful repairman who knows how to communicate and who is happy—that means everything to me."

Although it is vitally important to ensure all students have equal access and resources to pursue college if they so choose, it is equally important that we recognize, value, and support alternative paths to success that reflect the students' own interests and passions. A high school student named Alana shared with me:

> "I want to be happy with my job. I see everybody else in my family, and they're not happy in their jobs."

And speaking of being happy in your job . . . I recall a rather unique student success story of my own: Brandon's story. When I was a teacher, Brandon was a high school senior in my class. He was labeled E.D. (emotionally disturbed). I found him to be bright, funny, sensitive, and sweet. A few years after Brandon graduated, he called me, excited to share his news. He had landed his dream job. "That's wonderful," I told Brandon, "What are you doing?" "I pick up dead bodies for a mortuary." My heart sank. Maybe Brandon really is emotionally disturbed, I thought to myself. I cautiously asked Brandon to explain. Why did he consider this his dream job? He went on to explain that when he arrives to pick up a body, there are people there who are grieving the loss of a loved one. He explained how he's able to console them and treat their loved one with respect. This is the part of the job that Brandon loves—feeling like he's making a difference in people's lives when they are in pain. He is able to show them compassion and empathy. Hearing this, my heart soared once again for Brandon. I told him, "You know, not many people can do what you do and feel good about it." He said, "I know, but I can, and I'm good at it." He knew he had a special ability that many do not possess, and he felt proud and accomplished for it. As odd as his job choice may sound to others, we need more people like Brandon in this world.

These somewhat unconventional student success stories tell us the importance of nonacademic measures of educational growth, human development, and life-skill attainment as a priority of at least equal value to academics. Prioritizing and fostering SEL skill development is vital to the success of all individuals, regardless of the paths they choose beyond high school. That said, SEL can make a profound impact on student success along the path to higher education as well. Studies show that more often than not, students drop out of college due to social and emotional challenges more often than academic challenges. Additionally, students from marginalized populations often do not have the social and emotional support systems needed to pursue and sustain successful college careers. With high school counselors overburdened with unrealistic numbers of students assigned to them, in some states as high as 800 or more students per counselor, what measures can be taken to ensure kids have the information, guidance, and resources needed to pursue higher education and not fall through the cracks? Let's explore that question from the perspective of the students themselves.

Bill, an 18-year-old senior, reflected on the benefits of his small SEL-centered school environment over those of a larger school: "There's more kids at other schools, so they don't really have time to deal with every student individually. If they notice a student is upset, they can't really do anything because they have so many other students to worry about. Here, they actually care. They notice if someone is stuck on something [school work] or needs help. They notice if someone is upset."

Tony, also an 18-year-old senior, reflected on his positive relationship with one of his teachers, saying, "He's like a 10-years-older version of me," indicating that he found his teacher to be relatable to him and to his potential prospects in adulthood. Tony also shared with me that he might not be able to afford to go to college because, although he thinks the first two years are free, he is not sure about that because he doesn't have anyone in his family who went to college. He went on to say, "So, I might just get a job that doesn't really require college." One of Tony's suggestions for his school was to post "a big sign that says, 'How to Get into College.'" These student reflections are very telling as to the need and benefit of SEL-centered programming.

The Long-Term Impact of Expanding Student Horizons

According to Duckworth (2016), grit and growth mindset go hand in hand. Citing a study done in collaboration with Carol Dweck on over 2,000 high school seniors, Duckworth and Dweck discovered that the *grittiest,* or most resilient, students were those with a growth mindset. When students foresee limited options for their futures, intrinsic motivation to pursue and persist toward future goals is decreased. Increased options and the discovery of passion for a goal result in increased intrinsic motivation to persevere in attaining that goal.

This concept was revealed in my conversation with 19-year-old Jared-James, referenced in Chapter Two, in which he reflected on his people-watching observations while on a field trip to a metropolitan area. Although he did not know what those people wearing nice suits and driving expensive cars did for a living, he knew he wanted that for himself (intrinsic motivation). His comments also reflect a growth mindset: believing that he can grow in his ability to achieve and succeed and that it is within his own locus of control to do so (Dweck 2006).

Sally, a teacher, described an event that occurred during that same field trip, which included taking 21 teenagers on an overnight trip to a neighboring city for their leadership council. She went on to discuss what she feels was a significant event in the growth and development of her students' SEL skills. The students happened upon a lost little girl who had gotten separated from her mother, and the students explained to Sally that they witnessed many adults pass right by the little girl without any show of concern or attempt to help.

Sally was proud to report the way her students handled themselves in this situation. The students stopped to console the lost child and intervened to successfully reunite her with her mother. Sally describes the "attitude" of the students as, "We're going to do this. . . . We're going to be caring. . . . We're going to be leaders." Sally reflected on this display of empathy and leadership as "a magical moment." She stated that because it is an expectation for these students to practice and apply such SEL skills, the students in turn "deliver on that expectation." This speaks to the importance of adults expressing high expectations for students in how they conduct themselves in society. This gives students an opportunity to rise to the occasion and to see themselves in a different light. There is an important distinction to be made between being compassionate and understanding of students from marginalized populations and having low expectations for those students. The phrase, *the soft bigotry of low expectations* comes to mind.

Much consensus exists among educators, researchers, and policy makers in support of SEL, including emerging support for grit. Support for developing SEL among at-risk students is also found in the resiliency research, which cites mastery of SEL skills, such as self-regulation and emotion management, as primary mitigating factors in overcoming the effects of adversity (Walsh 2015).

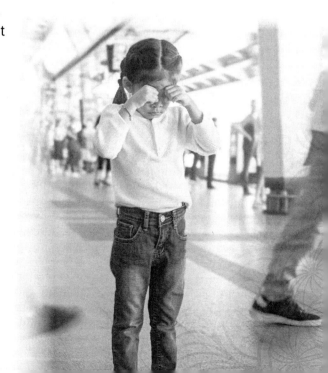

Altering the Trajectory of At-Risk Students

I'd like to share with you some personal reflections and anecdotal evidence as to the long-term impact SEL can have on student outcomes. The following are encounters I've had with three extraordinary young women whose lives are a testament to the power of SEL. Meet Taylor, Erica, and Jackie.

Persevering through Adversity: Taylor Penny

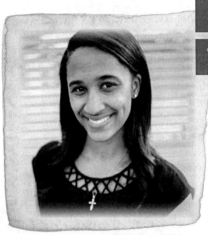

Taylor was raised by a loving and supportive single mother who strived to provide for her and her siblings. Taylor's mom sought the support of the local after-school program to help meet the family's needs, yet she remained a constant presence in advocating for Taylor's success. It was in the after-school program that Taylor established relationships with other caring adults who mentored her in all aspects of her life, of which there were many ups and downs. Beyond academic support, the staff provided Taylor with the additional social and emotional support she needed to be successful. They also assisted Taylor with the college application and financial aid process, which made it possible for her to apply to several colleges. Still, there were many times when the staff wondered whether she would "make it." She did make it. Taylor now credits the caring staff at her after-school program, along with the love and support of her family, for her ultimate success. She graduated from Washington State University in 2016 with a bachelor's degree, and she earned a master's degree from the University of Phoenix in 2018. Like many first-generation college students, assistance with the college application and financial aid process is crucial to their success. Lucky for Taylor, her mom encouraged her to pursue a college education and sought out the additional support needed to ensure her success.

Taylor adds that in addition to her family, the staff in the after-school program she attended as a kid were responsible for teaching her many life lessons and "tips" she continues to use to this day. Her story has come full circle, as she is now working in the very after-school program she credits for her success. Now, she is passing on her wisdom and experience to all the other "young Taylors" in her program.

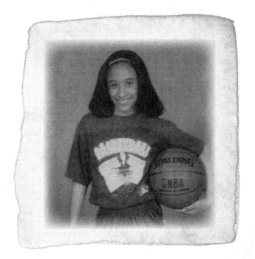

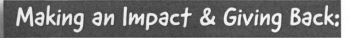

Making an Impact & Giving Back:

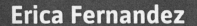

Erica Fernandez

Similar to Taylor, Erica also credits her after-school program and the SEL skills developed in that environment for her successful transition into college and adult life. Erica, along with her family, emigrated from Mexico to the United States at the age of 10. She was a serious and determined student from the start. Extremely bright and ambitious, she caught up academically and even surpassed her American-born counterparts quickly. Erica epitomized a growth mind-set, always wanting the most she could get out of her education. She expanded her learning time and opportunities by participating in the local after-school program.

Erica quickly became a leader among her peers, but she didn't stop there. As a teen, she discovered her passion for the environment and for the pursuit of social justice. She became a local community activist, leading the fight against a corporate effort that threatened an environmental concern for her low-socioeconomic community. Erica became a local hero while still in high school.

It is important to note that during the course of her high school career, Erica's family, who were migrant workers, had to relocate in search of work. Determined not to allow a move to disrupt her education, she opted to stay and finish high school. Erica was on her own, couch-surfing at various locations and, at one point, living in a friend's garage.

The social and emotional support she received from the caring adults in her life, including the staff at the after-school program, was instrumental in her ability to persevere toward her goals. Erica has since gone on to graduate from Stanford University and has worked for several organizations, including the U.S. Department of Education's Office for Civil Rights in Washington, D.C., in her pursuit of justice and equity. But she's not done yet. She plans to advance in both her education and her activism and to continue to give back to the community and to the country she feels gave her so much.

Erica's dedication to activism and community service is an incredible testament to cultivating SEL skills. I have no doubt we will be hearing much more about the great things she does in the future. Erica is the personification of *grit*.

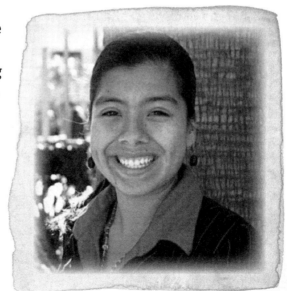

Finding Purpose and Relevancy:
Jackie Rotman

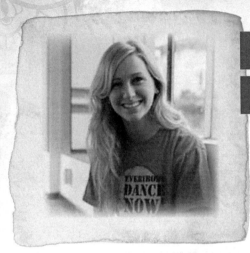

Jackie, like Erica, was a strong student academically, yet she struggled with identifying the relevance of what she was learning in school to her future. As Jackie puts it, "I felt frustrated that I was working so hard in school, but for what purpose? And I lacked a sense of direction for channeling my creativity and work ethic." Jackie found an outlet in dance. Fortunately for her, she came from a family that was able to provide her with the resources to access dance lessons in her after-school hours. Jackie discovered through dance that she was able to gain the social and emotional balance she needed to become a well-rounded and happy individual in addition to being a disciplined and driven student. But what she also realized at the young age of 12 was that not all students were as fortunate as she was in having the means to access extracurricular activities such as dance lessons. She recognized the opportunity gap. Young Jackie had something called *empathy*. She had the ability to recognize that other students could benefit from dance yet did not have the same access to it that she enjoyed.

She decided to do something about that, and in the process, found the meaning and relevancy she was searching for. Twelve-year-old Jackie started a nonprofit organization designed to bring SEL-infused dance activities to disadvantaged students in after-school programs. Jackie went on to pursue her academic goals, graduating from Stanford University (where she actually met Erica). She is now on her way to graduate school at Harvard University. Everybody Dance Now! (EDN), the nonprofit discussed in Chapter Four, is thriving with six chapters across the nation and with an intentional focus on cultivating SEL skills, such as confidence, self-esteem, and an appreciation for cultural diversity through dance.

What can be learned from these three stories, which are arguably the exception and not the norm? Making SEL a priority for all students can make stories like these the norm.

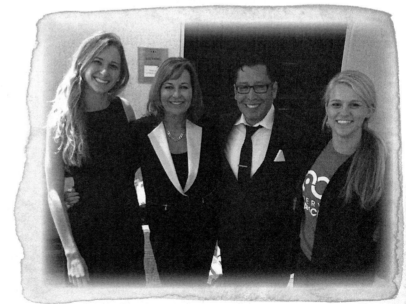

Summary

Educating students from a *whole-child* perspective is key and should be a priority in all K–12 educational policies and practices. SEL has the potential to mitigate inequities and narrow both the opportunity and achievement gaps by expanding students' horizons and equipping them with the social agency needed to navigate successfully into adulthood. The ultimate goal of education should be to produce well-rounded, well-adjusted, compassionate, engaged citizens who redefine the meaning of success.

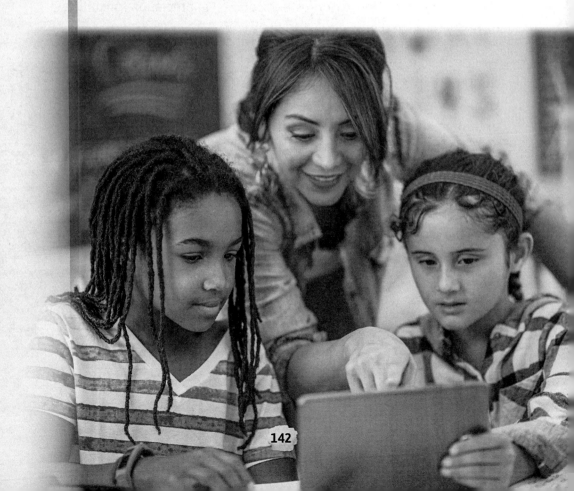

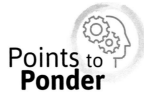

Points to Ponder

1. As you reflect on what you've read in this chapter and throughout the book, what are your thoughts and ideas about:

   » implementing SEL in your professional practice?

   » implementing SEL in your school, classroom, or program?

Points to **Ponder** *(cont.)*

2. What are your hopes and concerns for the future of SEL?

_____

_____

_____

_____

3. Do you have your own student success stories about the impact
   of SEL?

_____

_____

_____

_____

_____

_____

_____

_____

Appendix

References Cited

Afterschool Alliance. 2014. *America After 3PM: Afterschool Programs in Demand.* Washington, D.C.: Afterschool Alliance.

Barrett, Lisa Feldman. 2017. *How Emotions Are Made: The Secret Life of the Brain.* New York: First Mariner Books.

Bridgeland, John, and Mary Bruce. 2013. "The Missing Piece—How Social and Emotional Learning Can Empower Children and Transform Schools." *HuffPost.* Updated September 20, 2013. www.huffpost.com/entry/social-and-emotional -learning_b_3274283.

Bridgeland, John, Mary Bruce, and Arya Hariharan. 2013. *The Missing Piece: A National Teacher Survey on How Social and Emotional Learning Can Empower Children and Transform Schools.* Chicago: Collaborative for Academic, Social, and Emotional Learning.

California Department of Education. "Program Description." Updated June 11, 2018. www.cde.ca.gov/ls/ba/as/pgmdescription.asp.

California Department of Education, After School Division, and the California AfterSchool Network. 2014. *Quality Standards for Expanded Learning in California: Creating and Implementing a Shared Vision of Quality.* http://www .afterschoolnetwork.org/sites/main/files/file-attachments/quality_standards.pdf.

Collaborative for Academic, Social, and Emotional Learning (CASEL). 2015. *2015 CASEL Guide: Effective Social and Emotional Learning Programs—Middle and High School Ed.* secondaryguide.casel.org.

———. 2017. "Core SEL Competencies." casel.org/core-competencies/.

———. "Federal Policy." Accessed June 15, 2018. casel.org/federal -policy-and-legislation/.

———. 2018. "State Scan Scorecard Project." casel.org/state-scan -scorecard-project-2/.

———. "What Is SEL?" Accessed June 15, 2018. casel.org/what-is-sel/.

Cranston, Amy. 2017. "Want to Know the Secret to Prioritizing School Climate?" *Leadership* 46, no. 5 (May/June 2017).

Cranston, Bryan. 2016. *A Life in Parts.* New York: Scribner.

Davis, Jeff. 2015. *State of the State of Expanded Learning in California 2014–2015.*

California AfterSchool Network. http://www.afterschoolnetwork.org/sites/main/files/file-attachments/state_of_the_state_of_expanded_learning_in_ca_2014-14.pdf.

DePaoli, Jennifer L., Matthew N. Atwell, and John Bridgeland. 2017. *Ready to Lead: A National Principal Survey on How Social and Emotional Learning Can Prepare Children and Transform Schools*. Washington, DC: Civic Enterprises and Hart Research Associates.

Duckworth, Angela. 2016. *Grit: The Power of Passion and Perseverance*. New York: Scribner.

Dweck, Carol S. 2006. *Mindset: The New Psychology of Success*. New York: Ballantine Books.

Elias, Maurice J., and Harriet Arnold, eds. 2006. *The Educator's Guide to Emotional Intelligence and Academic Achievement: Social-Emotional Learning in the Classroom*. Thousand Oaks, CA: Corwin Press.

Fulghum, Robert. 1986. *All I Really Need to Know, I Learned in Kindergarten*. New York: Ballantine Books.

Gardner, Howard. 1983. *Frames of Mind: The Theory of Multiple Intelligences*. New York: Basic Books.

———. 2006. *Multiple Intelligences: New Horizons*. New York: Basic Books.

Goleman, Daniel. 1995. *Emotional Intelligence: Why It Can Matter More than IQ*. New York: Bantam Books.

———. 2006. *Social Intelligence: The New Science of Human Relationships*. New York: Bantam Books.

Herman, Keith C., Jal'et Hickmon-Rosa, and Wendy M. Reinke. 2017. "Empirically Derived Profiles of Teacher Stress, Burnout, Self-Efficacy, and Coping and Associated Student Outcomes." *Journal of Positive Behavior Interventions* 20, no. 2: 90–100.

Hollie, Sharroky. 2018. *Culturally and Linguistically Responsive Teaching and Learning, 2nd Ed*. Huntington Beach, CA: Teacher Created Materials.

Jensen, Eric. 2009. *Teaching with Poverty in Mind: What Being Poor Does to Kids' Brains and What Schools Can Do About It*. Alexandria, VA: ASCD.

Jones, Damon, Daniel Max Crowley, and Mark Greenberg. 2017. "Improving Social Emotional Skills in Childhood Enhances Long-Term Well-Being and Economic Outcomes." Edna Bennet Pierce Prevention Research Center, Pennsylvania State University.

Jones, Damon E., Mark Greenberg, and Max Crowley. 2015. "Early Social-Emotional

Functioning and Public Health: The Relationship Between Kindergarten Social Competence and Future Wellness." *American Journal of Public Health* 105, no. 11: 2283–2290.

Jones, Stephanie, Katharine Brush, Rebecca Bailey, Gretchen Brion-Meisels, Joseph McIntyre, Jennifer Kahn, Bryan Nelson, and Laura Stickle. 2017. *Navigating SEL from the Inside Out: Looking Inside and Across 25 Leading SEL Programs: A Practical Resource for Schools and OST Providers (Elementary School Focus).* Cambridge, MA: Harvard Graduate School of Education.

Kielburger, Craig, Holly Branson, and Marc Kielburger. 2018. *WEconomy: You Can Find Meaning, Make a Living, and Change the World.* Hoboken, NJ: John Wiley and Sons, Inc.

Leroy, Carol, and Brent Symes. 2001. "Teachers' Perspectives on the Family Backgrounds of Children at Risk." *McGill Journal of Education* 36, no. 1.

Luthar, Suniya S. 2003. "The Culture of Affluence: Psychological Costs of Material Wealth." Child Development 74, no. 6 (November 2003): 1581–1593. Accessed August 17, 2007. https://doi.org/10.1046/j.1467-8624.2003.00625.x.

McLeod, Saul. n.d. "Maslow's Hierarchy of Needs." *Simply Psychology.* Updated 2018. http://www.simplypsychology.org/maslow.html.

Miyamoto, Koji. 2015. "The Global Search for Education: New Study—Social and Emotional Learning," interview by C. M. Rubin. *The Huffington Post.* Updated December 6, 2017. www.huffingtonpost.com/c-m-rubin/the-global-search-for -edu_b_7108336.html.

National Center for Missing & Exploited Children (NCMEC). 2019. "Child Sex Trafficking." www.missingkids.com/theissues/trafficking.

———. 2018. "NCMEC and Honeywell Team Up to Fight Sexual Abuse through Education," news release, August 27, 2018, https://www .prnewswire.com/news-releases/ncmec-and-honeywell-team-up -to-fight-child-sexual-abuse-through-education-300702681.html.

O'Neil, Michelle. 2018. "Collateral Damage: New Immigration Policies and Education in California." *Learning in Afterschool & Summer.* http://blog.learninginafterschool .org/2018/07/collateral-damage-new-immigration.html.

Partnership for Children and Youth and the Expanded Learning 360/365 Project. 2015. *Student Success Comes Full Circle: Leveraging Expanded Learning Opportunities.*

Pittman, Karen. n.d. "SEL, Whole Child Education, and Student Readiness: How Do They Connect?" AASA, Updated July 20, 2017.aasa.org/totalchild.aspx?id=41408 &blogid=83505.

Puddicombe, Andy. 2011. *The Headspace Guide to Meditation & Mindfulness.* New York: St. Martin's Press.

Rumberger, Russell W., and Sun Ah Lim. 2008. *Why Students Drop Out of School: A Review of 25 Years of Research*. California Dropout Research Project. Santa Barbara, CA: Gevirtz Graduate School of Education.

Sandy Hook Advisory Commission. 2015. *Final Report of the Sandy Hook Advisory Commission*, 110–111.

SEL Solutions. 2015. "Are You Ready to Assess Social and Emotional Development?" Washington, D.C.: American Institutes for Research.

Smith, Charles, Gina McGovern, Reed Larson, Barbara Hillaker, and Stephen C. Peck. 2016. *Preparing Youth to Thrive: Promising Practices for Social & Emotional Learning*. Washington, D.C.: Forum for Youth Investment.

Smith, Tracey. 2018. "10 Ways We Made Our School Happier," eSchool News, June 7, 2018. www.eschoolnews.com/2018/06/07/10-ways-we-made-our-school -happier/.

Sportel, Brandon. 2015. "How to Turn Elementary School Teachers into Emotional Detectives," *Time*, May 27, 2015. time.com/3897741/elementary-school-teacher -bullying-protect/.

Steinberg, Laurence. 2015. "How Self-Control Drives Student Achievement." *Educational Leadership* 73, no. 2: 28–32. Alexandria, VA: ASCD.

Supporting Emotional Learning Act, H.R. 497, 114th Congress (2015). https://www .congress.gov/bill/114th-congress/house-bill/497.

Tough, Paul. 2012. *How Children Succeed: Grit, Curiosity, and the Hidden Power of Character*. New York: Houghton Mifflin Harcourt.

Walsh, Bari. 2015. "The Science of Resilience: Why Some Children Can Thrive Despite Adversity." Harvard Graduate School of Education. https://www.gse.harvard.edu /news/uk/15/03/science-resilience.

Zernike, Kate. 2016. "Testing for Joy and Grit? Schools Nationwide Push to Measure Students' Emotional Skills." *New York Times*, February 29, 2016. http://www .nytimes.com/2016/03/01/us/testing-for-joy-and-grit-schools-nationwide-push -to-measure-students-emotional-skills.html.

Zinshteyn, Mikhail. 2015. "What Does It Mean to Have 'Grit' in the Classroom?" *The Atlantic*, July 23, 2015. http://www.theatlantic.com/education/archive/2015/07 /what-grit-looks-like-in-the-classroom/399197/.

Recommended Reading

SEL Research and Theory

Handbook of Social and Emotional Learning: Research and Practice (Durlak, et al. 2015).

How Emotions Are Made: The Secret Life of the Brain (Barrett 2018).

The Marshmallow Test: Why Self-Control is the Engine of Success (Mischel 2014).

Mindset: The New Psychology of Success (Dweck 2006).

Multiple Intelligences: New Horizons (Gardner 2006).

The Well-Managed Classroom: Strategies to Create a Productive and Cooperative Social Climate in Your Learning Community (Hensley et al. 2007).

SEL Assessment, Implementation, and Practice

Aha! Method Book: Socially and Emotionally Intelligent Approach to Working with Teenagers (Freed 2016).

Helping Children Succeed: What Works and Why (Tough 2016).

PeaceQ: Increasing the Capacity for Peace Within and Peace Beyond (Freed 2016).

Promoting Grit, Tenacity, and Perseverance: Critical Factors for Success in the 21st Century (U.S. Department of Education 2013).

Meditation and Mindfulness

The Headspace Guide to Meditation & Mindfulness (Puddicombe 2015).

Project-Based Learning

The Educator's Guide to Emotional Intelligence and Academic Achievement: Social-Emotional Learning in the Classroom (Elias and Arnold 2006).

Preparing Youth to Thrive: Promising Practices for Social and Emotional Learning. (Smith et al. 2016).

Service Learning

The Educator's Guide to Emotional Intelligence and Academic Achievement: Social-Emotional Learning in the Classroom (Elias and Arnold 2006).

WEconomy: You Can Find Meaning, Make a Living, and Change the World (Kielburger, Branson, and Kielburger 2018).

At-Risk Students

Culturally and Linguistically Responsive Teaching and Learning: Classroom Practices for Student Success. Second Edition (Hollie 2018).

Don't Call Them Dropouts: Understanding the Experiences of Young People Who Leave High School before Graduation (America's Promise Alliance 2014).

Emotional Poverty in All Demographics: How to Reduce Anger, Anxiety and Violence in the Classroom (Payne 2018).

Engaging Students with Poverty in Mind: Practical Strategies for Raising Achievement (Jensen 2013).

I Wish My Teacher Knew: How One Question Can Change Everything for Our Kids (Schwartz 2016).

Teaching with Poverty in Mind: What Being Poor Does to Kids' Brains and What Schools Can Do About It (Jensen 2009).

Things I Wish My Teacher Knew About Me: Memoir of a Disengaged Student (Matthews 2015).

Why Students Drop Out of School: A Review of 25 Years of Research (Rumberger and Lim 2008).

Family Engagement

Beyond the Bake Sale: The Essential Guide to Family-School Partnerships (Henderson et al. 2007).

Principles & Parables: Correspondence Between Grandfather & Grandson (Seidman and Miller 2016).

Resource List

SEL Research, Policy, Assessment and Implementation Tools

American Institutes for Research (AIR): **www.air.org**

Aspen Institute: **www.aspeninstitute.org**

The Big EQ Campaign: **www.bigeqcampaign.org**

CASEL: **www.casel.org**

Committee for Children: **www.cfchildren.org**

CORE Districts: **www.coredistricts.org**

The Forum for Youth Investment: **www.forumfyi.org**

The Greater Good Science Center at the University of California, Berkeley: **www.greatergood.berkeley.edu**

Making Caring Common Project at Harvard Graduate School of Education: **www.mcc.gse.harvard.edu/resources-by-topic/social-emotional-learning**

Mindful Schools: **www.mindfulschools.org**

National Center for School Mental Health: **csmh.umaryland.edu**

Partnership for Children and Youth (PCY): **www.partnerforchildren.org**

SEL4US: **www.sel4us.org**

Six Seconds: **www.6seconds.org**

U.S. Department of Education: **www.ed.gov**

Yale Center for Emotional Intelligence: **www.ei.yale.edu**

SEL Curriculum and Programming

Brandon Sportel's article: **www.zocalopublicsquare.org/2015/05/26/how-to-turn-elementary-school-teachers-into-emotional-detectives/ideas/nexus**

EduCare Foundation: **www.educarefoundation.com**

Edutopia: **www.edutopia.org/social-emotional-learning**

Everybody Dance Now! (EDN): **www.everybodydancenow.org**

Headspace: **www.headspace.com**

HelloYello: **www.helloyello.net**

MindUP: **www.mindup.org**

National Center for Missing and Exploited Children: **missingkids.org**

Playing Field Foundation: **www.playingfieldfoundation.org**

Sanford Harmony: **www.sanfordharmony.org**

Second Step: **www.secondstep.org**

Temescal Associates: **www.temescalassociates.com**

The First Tee: **www.thefirsttee.org**

U.S. Soccer Foundation: **www.ussoccerfoundation.org**

WE Schools: **www.we.org/we-schools**

WINGS for Kids: **www.wingsforkids.org**

Write Brain Books: **www.writebrainbooks.com**